REQUIEM FOR A GREAT KILLER

Other books by Harley Williams

Imagination

Northern Lights and Western Stars
The Inheritors
Fingal's Box
At Cape Faithful

Biographical Portraits

Doctors Differ
The Healing Touch
Between Life and Death
The Conquest of Fear
Three Men of Stress
Don Quixote of the Microscope
Great Biologists

Criticism

A Doctor Looks at Miracles

Educational

Your Heart

Requiem for a Great Killer

The story of Tuberculosis

by Harley Williams

Health Horizon London

Published by Health Horizon Limited for
The Chest and Heart Association
Tavistock House North, London, WC1
and printed by Waterlow London

ISBN 0 901548 32 4

CONTENTS

Dedication

To the many whose lives were marred by
the killer . . . especially one whose
life touched mine but whom I never saw.

AUTHOR'S PREFACE

My involvement in this theme began when I became a medical student at Edinburgh University. Not only in my first year, but on the very first day. The courses had not started and I had no one to talk to. Coming out of a bookshop, after buying Cunningham's *Manual of Practical Anatomy*, and having the intense curiosity of the novice about what might be going on, I sauntered idly across to the University hall, where a lecture of some kind was just about to begin. In such a mood I was ready to hear about any subject under the sun. Newly appointed professors used to deliver the inaugural lecture in public, and here was I at the back of the hall, listening to a new teacher, who spoke professorially for the first time.

That professor was Sir Robert Philip, and the subject of his inaugural lecture was Tuberculosis.

Hippocrates the father of medicine said that in Time there is much Opportunity. But in Opportunity there is little Time. Some power – not myself – made me embrace the opportunity, and since that fateful day I have been immersed in this fascinating and terrible subject.

This is not a textbook nor is it addressed mainly to doctors. The specialists will not find here what they can easily discover in works of reference. In fact, this is not the description of a disease at all. It is the human story of man's enterprise in the conquest of an illness which has probably touched more lives than any other. And the killer is not yet killed.

In this 'Requiem' for those who have suffered and died and the physicians and nurses who have dedicated their lives to cure, the note of sadness proper to a "Requiem" dissolves into a paean of triumph.

ACKNOWLEDGMENTS

Dr. J. Greenwood Wilson has shown enormous enthusiasm for this book and he has revised the text critically and made numerous constructive suggestions. Without his help it would not have been what it has become.

Dr. Norman Lloyd Rusby has placed his great medical knowledge at my disposal. He has read the whole book and enabled many mistakes to be eliminated. I am greatly indebted to him.

Dr. James Parrish, expert bacteriologist and historian of medicine, has carefully scrutinised these chapters, supplied many helpful ideas and corrected errors.

Mrs. Mary Wells has re-typed the manuscript, not once but several times most conscientiously.

Chapter 1

The Killer Before the Dawn

ON many a hot Mediterranean hillside two thousand years ago, a gilt statue of the god Aesculapius, patron of healing, would be found in a thick grove of pine and myrtle. There in the shade of the trees was his temple and his circle of physicians and apprentices. Near at hand was a healing spring, and twining themselves around the marble columns a few snakes were kept for ornamental purposes. All along the ancient Mediterranean shore, the doctors were ultimately pupils of Hippocrates the Father of Medicine and his successor Galen. Among patients waiting in these temple-surgeries were many with a disease called phthisis. They sat on the marble benches coughing, short of breath. Sometimes they had blood-spitting which the Greeks called haemoptysis – a word we still use today. The physicians treated them with honey diluted with wine barley gruel, dark resinous wine mixed with water, and herbs grown in the temple garden. The leading Mediterranean doctors were usually Greeks, and they travelled from city to city wearing purple robes and gold belts and laurel wreaths round their long hair, and they carried with them the books of Hippocrates on sheepskin scrolls. These nomadic physicians were flexible and opportunist. Often they advised their phthisical patients to take water from the local spring. On the slopes of Mount Vesuvius, sulphur fumes from the volcano were considered beneficial. There was one Graeco-Arabian sage who recommended a mixture of red roses and honey. Goat's milk was a frequent favourite. Wherever they went, they met cases of phthisis, for it was man's terrible companion, half domesticated, half savage, a killer which appeared out of nowhere and behaved in a manner incomprehensible to the best doctors of the day, however great their professional pretensions. So through many centuries Greek knowledge endured and Greek books were translated into Arabic, then Latin and the tradition came to England. William Shakespeare knew about Phthisis, and in his day one out of every five deaths in London were caused by it. Our King Charles II is said to have touched with his royal hand some ninety thousand patients suffering from the glandular form of the disease – Scrofula – with reputedly good results.

By the end of the eighteenth century the doctors were still reading the text books of Galen, the Greek of the first century, who had systematised the Hippocratic doctrines. Every kind of remedy was being tried: goat's milk, sea bathing, wine and gruel, horse riding, bleeding, washing in the sacred spring, cod liver oil . . . . The remedies remained constant within variety – constant in their ineffectiveness. The patient went on coughing and wasting away, panting along his road to a premature death. In the Industrial Revolution, the fatalities from phthisis mounted to a peak.

Only at the end of the nineteenth century, almost within living memory, did there come a momentous break in the darkness, and the modern story of tuberculosis can well begin at the very end of the Victorian age.

In 1898, out of 36,000,000 people who lived in Britain, 70,000 lives were lost through tuberculosis. In 1948, half a century later, the deaths were less than 27,000 although meanwhile the population had risen to 48,000,000. This remarkable change represents a saving of a million and a half lives, and on the computation that for every death there were five to ten persons ill from tuberculosis, the relief in human suffering must have affected five or ten million individuals. How was this notable revolution achieved?

2

On Tuesday, 20th December, 1898, in the drawing room of Marlborough House, London, the personal residence of

H.R.H. The Prince of Wales, there was born an organisation called 'The National Association for the Prevention of Consumption and other forms of Tuberculosis'. On this day the world heard the words of a future king "if preventable, why not prevented?" In that dignified atmosphere of gilt, portraits and chandeliers, the gentlemen wore frock coats and we can be sure that the speeches were measured and dignified. They were what would now be called 'top people'. The presiding figure is of course His Royal Highness but gathered around him are the Marquis of Salisbury, Lord Rosebery, the Earl of Derby and prominent men from the two political parties, also from the church, the universities and commerce, and with them some eminent physicians: Sir William Broadbent, Bart., Sir Samuel Wilks, Bart., Sir James Crichton-Browne, Sir Thomas Grainger Stewart from Edinburgh and Dr. John Moore from Dublin.

At this distance of time it is hard to measure what brought together this group of diverse human beings, men of affairs, lawyers and bankers, and frock-coated doctors. Most of them can have known little about the subject, but they were intrigued by its novelty, and of course impressed to be invited to Marlborough House. The physicians among them were about to do what was seldom done before – discuss medical matters in public and invite the layman to take a part in conquering a disease. That ancient curse called consumption was now, according to the physicians, caused by an invisible microbe. The Prince himself was on the verge of sixty. He had lost his father the Prince Consort from typhoid fever and he himself had successfully passed through the same illness as a young man. His Coronation as Edward VII was to be delayed by an attack of appendicitis, and he made medical history in being one of the first patients in whom the appendix was successfully removed. Perhaps he felt he owed something to the medical profession. Members of that distinguished audience were prepared to follow such eminent leadership into strange country. Even the famous doctors were far from being unanimous about consumption. The discovery of the germ in 1882 had not carried treatment very far forward, and a vaccine called tuberculin which had been proposed as a cure was a disappointment. Great movements are often born like this – against a background of doubt and mistrust. However The National Association was duly formed, and its aims defined in a splendid sentence. "The mission of a newly formed body was to carry into every dwelling in the land an elementary knowledge of the mode in which consumption is propagated and of the means by which its spread may be prevented and thus to strengthen the hands of medical men throughout the country who are dealing with individual cases of the disease." To capture public imagination, arouse the self-protective instincts of the public, eliminate tuberculosis in cattle, encourage sanatoria for open-air treatment. This was the programme, and the methods would be through instruction and persuasion, not compulsion. The President of the Royal College of Physicians (Sir Samuel Wilks) duly moved the setting up of an influential committee, of which the Prince was President, and the Earl of Derby, Chairman. With the hindsight of seventy years we may judge that these solemn aspirations which seemed so bold, were modest indeed, but an important step had been taken, and the gracious act on the part of the Prince in calling the meeting in his own home would save hundreds of thousands of lives. The obstacles were formidable. The Royal College of Physicians was lukewarm, fearing that panic would be created by talking about an infectious disease. Some dreaded the thought of compulsory notification and restrictive legislation.

One man alone had power to wave the magic wand which overcame this opposition. It was Sir William Broadbent, the Prince's personal physician. He was written off by his medical brethren as an impulsive crusader, but fortunately he was not a man to wait for everyone's approval before throwing himself into the idea. Great movements originate in the individual, and to Sir William Broadbent the credit can be given for the start of an antituberculosis movement in Britain.

He was a Yorkshireman, apprenticed to a doctor in Manchester before going up to St. George's Hospital, London. He passed his final in the year 1859 and settled down in practice in the

West End where he had the usual struggle to make ends meet. He became physician to St. Mary's Hospital in 1861 and thereafter moved up rapidly in the world. In 1892 he went to live in Brook Street, a more fashionable address, and was soon the Prince's Physician-In-Ordinary. Sir William was now a very busy man who saved time over lunch by eating a rice pudding in his carriage. He wrote all his professional letters with his own pen and never dictated. When he retired from his post as physician to St. Mary's he had even more time to give to the antituberculosis movement.

Just as a Prince can be inspired by his Physician-In-Ordinary, so that physician can be set on fire by another less prominent but well-informed specialist. I guess that Sir William Broadbent had been brought in to the movement by an equally dynamic physician who became Sir Malcolm Morris (1849–1924).

3

Malcom Morris had graduated from St. Mary's and after postgraduate work in Berlin and Vienna became a skin specialist. In his practice syphilis would play a large part. In this disease there was then no specific treatment, and a large area was left to clinical judgement. Malcolm Morris was over thirty when he heard of Robert Koch's discovery of the TB germ, and actually witnessed an exhibition of staining of the organism which was to the doctors of that era almost the equivalent of a space landing today. Morris had a gift for communication and became editor of *The Practitioner* (still flourishing seventy years after). His editorial in June 1898 must have had something to do with the support which this antituberculosis campaign aroused among doctors. Malcolm Morris painted a bold picture. Tuberculosis was ubiquitous – in the strictest meaning of that word – and only deserts and mountain ranges were exempt from its attacks. Consumption caused the deaths of about one eleventh of the population in Great Britain, and in the whole of Europe the mortality was not less than one million every year. No pestilence in history had made anything like the havoc wrought by tuberculosis, and when in addition to the destruction of life, human suffering is taken into account, tuberculosis was one of the worst afflictions of the human race. Malcolm Morris appealed for a leader – a Peter the Hermit* – to start a crusade. This was indeed a holy cause.

Despite the high mortality, tuberculosis had in fact decreased by two thirds over the last half of the nineteenth century and a prospect was that the next thirty years would see its disappearance. The number of consumptives who could be cured by treatment was already four times what it had been at the beginning of the century. Many famous men whose careers were threatened by this disease in youth had lived on to be old men. One survivor of Napoleon's army who was invalided after Waterloo as a helpless consumptive had recently died at the highly respectable age of 103. At the present time, continued Malcolm Morris, not less than a quarter of a million people suffered from tuberculosis in Britain and only a very small proportion had no hope of cure. "Let us have a national crusade against a national disease", he preached. Malcolm Morris went on with his skin diseases and was also a well-known writer and speaker. He believed the secret of keeping young was to cultivate an interest in movements for the betterment of one's fellow men.

The first public effort of the new Association was to set up the British Congress on Tuberculosis which was held in 1901. This was an enormous success and Robert Koch himself came over from Berlin. Meanwhile the Association formed branches throughout the country and held its first annual meeting with Dr. St. Clair Thomson as Secretary of the Organising Committee. He was himself a victim of tuberculosis who became a famous laryngologist. The first drops of a cataract of educational literature came forth. In its first year the office expenses of running the Organisation were some £293, and £760 was in the bank.

However the shadow of conformity still brooded over this

* *A French monk of the eleventh century who inspired the first crusade.*

promising new venture. The Prime Minister, Lord Salisbury, "deprecated any appeal to legislative interference." But the Committee expressed itself to the contrary. "In some respects an occasional mild dose of legislation might be of advantage in the furtherance of the object we have in hand." The Council brought pressure to bear on the Government. A noted speaker in those early debates was Professor Clifford Allbutt (Cambridge). He boldly asserted that Britain had lost the lead in the prevention of tuberculosis because English people had not enough faith in "theoretical studies" (e.g. Research) such as the work of Pasteur and Koch. Many advances in medicine have sprung from the "theoretical enquiries of students in laboratories and academies", and if we had in Britain more Chairs of Comparative Pathology "there was a discovery to be made every day before dinner" but other speakers would not admit that Britain had fallen behind. They said that on the contrary, England had led the way and a country which had reduced the death rate from tuberculosis in the way which had happened in this country had no reason to be ashamed. The Germans had followed our example, as was high time. This was too much for Professor Allbutt who made in his own vigorous style a stirring rejoinder.

Such were the first polemics which echoed for more than fifty years and which gave the antituberculosis movement a characteristically controversial flavour. Contrary opinions, vigorously expressed, are a sign of vitality, and the movement had certainly made a good start. Although we, at our safe distance, are surprised at the modesty of these men's objectives, we can hardly imagine the prodigious obstacles they faced. Tuberculosis caused an enormous mortality, yet according to Malcolm Morris, there were few cases that could not be cured. Clifford Allbutt praised German research, but other speakers asserted that we in this country had got much further without research! In Britain there were hardly any sanatoria and few specialised facilities. Yet the Prime Minister "deprecated legislative interference" – that is any action on the part of Government which would provide facilities beyond existing medical resources. We look back on these pioneers with admiration if we measure the grandeur of their aims against the poverty of their resources.

A few years after this the Association secured as its Chairman an aristocratic and charming personality, Sir Arthur Stanley, brother of the Earl of Derby, who had been one of the early founders. Sir Arthur had been in the diplomatic service, but had become gravely handicapped by arthritis which obliged him to walk with two sticks. He was Chairman of the Red Cross and House Governor of St. Thomas's Hospital, London, where he actually lived. As Chairman of the National Association he was an urbane and lively presence who drew support from many quarters and represented a strong current of typically English philanthropy and concern for the unfortunate.

The story of tuberculosis during the first half century is presented here with a voluntary organisation as the framework. Clearly, of course, our success in the campaign could not be due to any single cause: nor is it contended that the Association's influence achieved all that was in fact accomplished. However, the public interest, public knowledge, and public awareness as expressed through the Association's work is a good yardstick. And it reminds us that in preventing a disease nothing whatever will be achieved unless it has public approval behind it.

The intention of this book is to present tuberculosis not merely as a series of theoretical discoveries and administrative acts, but as a great catalyser in a human being's life, we may look at some of its greatest victims. Their case histories gain interest from their accomplishments, but in essence show that genius must meet the same danger common to thousands.

Chapter 2

Victims of the Great White Scourge

THIS dreadful thing was generally known as the Great White Scourge, or a 'decline', or 'consumption' – vague terms to describe a dark phobia. It came into the family, and once cough and wasting had begun, it would continue its frightful course for months and years. Look at memorial notices in churchyards of the last century and you can picture the sad histories of young people, infants, adolescents and young adults who perished in this way. Whenever it appeared, the family foresaw an exhausting fight, with occasional remissions and probably a fatal end. But we hear only of the fatalities we do not hear of those who recovered.

Part of the legend is that consumption was a special enemy of genius, and of brokenhearted lovers, and it is even suggested that the disease was the source of the genius. Some have theorised that the toxin of consumption produced a heightened sensibility of the imagination, a febrile brilliance which created the poet and the artist. Can this genius theory be supported? Should we agree that those heroic consumptives whose poetry and music we still enjoy owed their talents to nothing but a bacillus and its toxins? It is interesting to take a new look at some outstanding artists whose lives were moulded by this malady.

One penetrating critic, Middleton Murry, believed that the genius which died with William Shakespeare in 1616 reappeared for a few short years in John Keats. He came to manhood in the age when Europe had just thrown off the tyrant Napoleon. He reached his splendid maturity when Europe was weary. He was a neat, thick-set youth, only five feet tall, with a singular charm of personality. He lived comfortably upon a small income left by his father and at the age of 16 was apprenticed to a local surgeon-apothecary and worked at filling bottles, cleaning bowls, scrubbing instruments. Later he walked the wards at Guy's Hospital, a conscientious though not dedicated student, and by the time he took his diploma at the Apothecaries' Hall in the year of Waterloo, John Keats had abandoned all idea of practising surgery. In the village of Hampstead on the edge of London he read poetry and enjoyed a convivial life with the liberal spirits of the age, always a good humoured companion who kept his miseries hidden under an iron pride. John Keats was a poet in pure culture, not consumed with lust for foreign travel like Byron, and he had no itch to put humanity right, like Shelley. To his friends, Keats was supremely rare, and normally sane. They admired his verse but did not esteem it as highly as we do now.

The stress of living in peaceful Hampstead a century and a half ago was no less than today, for stress is always proportional to the sufferer's sensibility. Keats lived the gracious life in days when a shilling was a fortune, and he had only to go on to the wild Hampstead Heath to hear the nightingale which we still hear in his poem. There was nothing neurotic about John Keats, yet he paid heavily for his creative moments. Some tuberculous patients are like that, enigmas to themselves and to those who know them best. Keats was a normal man though he had the ambition to be a great poet.

At 23 he went on a walking tour with his friend Brown to the Scottish Highlands. They reached the Isle of Mull, saw the cathedral of Iona and Fingal's Cave and returned to London by ship from Inverness. It was a wonderful holiday but for Keats it was the beginning of the end. That tour exhausted him. He shocked a friend by appearing at her house "with scarcely any shoes left, his jacket all torn at the back, a fur cap, a great plaid and his knapsack."

That same year John Keats met a certain Mrs. Brawne, and Mrs. Brawne had a daughter, Fanny. At this same critical moment in his life, his younger brother Tom, to whom he was devoted, died after a wasting illness of a few weeks during which John was both doctor and nurse. Meanwhile he wrote love letters to Fanny Brawne who was flattered by his attentions but quite unaware that her lover was a special sort of person. She had no idea how to assuage his inward wretchedness expressed in those passionate pages. Those love letters are indeed terrible in their tortured frenzy. All we know of Fanny Brawne is that she was unable to comprehend either his passion, or the malaise which was gradually stealing over John Keats. On a day in 1820 his friend Brown saw him walk into a room in a state of what seemed furious intoxication. Keats had taken a chill when sitting on the outside of the stage-coach between London and Hampstead. His friend put him to bed, and on touching the cold sheets, even before his head was on the pillow, Keats gave a cough and said "There is blood in my mouth . . . bring me a candle and let me see this blood." An apothecary knew how to recognise blood when he saw it, and he said to Brown with complete calm, "I cannot be deceived in the colour. That drop of blood is my death warrant. I must die." It is terrible to read that in this crisis the surgeon took away further blood from John Keats, and there was no idea of rest or hygiene. The poet knew better than anyone that his life was now to be measured in months. In those last two years came his greatest poetry. *The Grecian Urn: The Nightingale: Ode to Melancholy;* those poems are as fresh today as when he wrote them, but at the time they found no particular audience, and he certainly got no admiration from Mistress Brawne. Keats was advised to take the standard medical treatment that was offered to the phthisical patient – to live abroad. He wrote "There is no doubt that an English winter would put an end to me, and do so in a lingering, hateful manner. Therefore I must voyage or journey to Italy as a soldier marches up to a battery." The horrible thought of this journey haunted him each morning of his life. He was able to borrow money from painter friends, and left London by ship in the middle of September. After a tedious delay of six weeks in Naples for quarantine, he then reached Rome. In these last weeks no consumptive could have been more fortunate in his friend. Keats had Joseph Severn who volunteered to look after him and did so with touching fidelity. They lived, as everyone knows, in a house on the Spanish Steps. It was lucky that in Rome was a Scottish physician, Dr. James Clark (afterwards physician to Queen

Victoria) who was very kind to him. This was the same man whose unusual professional destiny it was to attend not only John Keats, but Frédéric Chopin and Robert Louis Stevenson.

There in the house on the Spanish Steps Keats suffered terrible relapses although occasionally he could walk in the Pincio Gardens. He became finicky in his food and once threw dishes out of the window. The two friends would take horse rides among the antiquities of Rome, but their peace was broken by violent, distressing fevers and repeated haemorrhages. Keats begged Severn to give him a bottle of laudanum to end his life, but Severn refused. The patient ate less and less and passed into a heavy delirium, though there were moments when Severn and even Dr. Clark took an optimistic view. For the last three weeks his friend never left the sick bed. This young man of 26, one of our very greatest poets, died miserably, without hope, or religion, or philosophy, or love. The unfortunate Severn had to pay £150 because all the bedding and furniture was burned through fear of infection.

Two years after her lover's death, Fanny Brawne married; she said about Keats, "The kindest thing to his memory would be to let it die" and she sold the ivory miniature of the poet's face.

2

On one of those great feudal estates in Poland that were really small kingdoms, François Frédéric Chopin was born to a Polish lady of peasant origin and a Frenchman who had got left behind in Napoleon's invasion. The country was Catholic, war stricken, and constantly harassed, by Napoleon, or the Germans, and especially by Russia. Chopin's music came from a mixture in himself of opposite cultures, the French and the Slav, and his genius was a spontaneous, natural thing. The music of his twenties is as fine as the compositions at the end. He was a thin, delicate boy who had to be coddled, and was sometimes sent for 'water cures', and when he was seventeen his younger sister died of acute phthisis. Supported by an admiring father, Chopin gave piano recitals all over Europe in the days when music was the prerogative of the salon. In the great houses of the Boulevard St. Germain, he had numerous pupils, and there were many love affairs but no marriage. He poured forth effortlessly those mazourkas, scherzos, and ballades which are still the main romantic glory of the piano. At twenty-five he had the first spitting of blood, but this was not thought to be a sign of consumption. Such a highly sensitive and ailing man was now taken in hand by a woman who was his complete opposite, who did not belong to the aristocratic salons, but came from the people, an atheist, a republican. This was the masculine Georges Sand who assumed control of Chopin's life. They went to the island of Majorca where they stayed in a gloomy Carthusian monastery. Chopin composed his twenty-four preludes against attacks of fever and it is interesting that his illness, although not properly diagnosed by the doctors, was greatly feared by those island peasants. As John Keats found in Rome, Chopin was shunned and was not even allowed a carriage to travel to catch the boat for Barcelona. He had to pay damages for his bed in the hotel which was burned afterwards. He had now what we should call obvious pulmonary tuberculosis, with attacks of shivering, coughing and spitting of blood, but still the doctors hesitated to give his illness that name. He was indeed unfortunate in his physicians. He continued to give those exquisite recitals, attend parties, and always charm the ladies, in an age when it was considered romantic for an artist to have a cough and occasionally spit blood. Then Chopin's father died – that father who always fostered his talent – and something went wrong with the young man's life. Georges Sand was twelve years older, a good nurse but too overpowering to live with, and the pious Catholic in Chopin recoiled from her rough agnosticism. He went to all kinds of doctors, even took the magnetic cure which was fashionable in Paris under Dr. Anton Mesmer. Eventually he separated from Georges Sand and in a year he would be dead. He fell in love with a young Countess, who belonged to one of the famous Polish houses, Delphine Potocka. There were two short visits to England where Chopin played before Queen Victoria, and even penetrated as far as a great county house of Keir in Perthshire which must have reminded him of Poland. I have actually played on the piano he used then. His last appearance in public was a London concert for Polish exiles, and afterwards he visited Dr. James Clark who had now returned from Rome to be Queen Victoria's physician – a kind man, but of limited understanding, who rejected the theory that consumption was infectious. Dr. Clark can have given Chopin little real hope. Then, back in Paris, and short of money, he consulted the well-known Dr. Pierre Louis who prescribed the singularly modern remedy of rest. Chopin gave a bitter answer: "Rest – I will have it soon without the doctors." There was an idea of sending him to the South of France, but he remained in Paris, and lived through an outbreak of Asiatic cholera. Delphine Potocka had a piano put into the sick room in the Place Vendôme and she sang to him while Chopin struggled to get his breath. He died at the age of thirty-nine.

He had enjoyed nineteen golden years to weave his magic enchantment. It is possible that rest and care, even without modern drugs could have prolonged his life without hampering his creativity, but it is doubtful. The delicate Chopin was more lucky in his illness than the robust John Keats.

3

The family of the Reverend Patrick Brontë, a Church of England clergyman living in a wild part of Yorkshire, is a terrible example of a medical history which was common at the beginning of the last century. The clergyman had one son and five girls who were sent to a Lancashire boarding school for the daughters of indigent clergymen. It was a shocking establishment, of the type that Charles Dickens satirised. The eldest girl Charlotte described the rigid discipline, the neglect, and the frequency of epidemics. Two or even four girls sometimes slept in one bed. In 1825 the school was swept by some kind of fever which may have been a virus infection, or an acute form of tuberculosis. Certainly two of the girls contracted consumption around this period and were brought home to die, the fatality being ascribed to the damp situation of the school. The brother Branwell who was touched with both genius and alcoholism died at thirty-one, and Emily Brontë who some believe the most gifted of the sisters, who wrote the novel *Wuthering Heights* died soon after. She had declined to see a doctor and was on her feet to the end. A younger sister Anne who wrote *The Tenant of Wildfell Hall* was sent to Scarborough for sea air and died of tuberculosis there. Then there was Charlotte, the eldest who had obviously the strongest resistance. She wrote her great book *Jane Eyre* and married a clergyman, but she died at thirty-nine as she was going to have a baby. The old father, the Reverend Patrick Brontë, lived on until eighty-four when he died from miscellaneous conditions among which was bronchitis.

Could there be a more vivid summary of an epidemic of family tuberculosis at the beginning of the 19th century?

4

In the old city of Edinburgh a tall young man with long hair used to walk up the hill to the Advocates' Library and the Law Courts. Robert Louis Stevenson was the only child of an engineer who had built lighthouses all around Scotland and who hoped that his boy would build more. Alas R.L.S. (as he had started to call himself) was devoted to the idea of becoming a writer but under his father's pressure agreed unwillingly to pass the examinations for the Scottish Bar. He was twenty-five when he was called to be an advocate, and he appeared in Court once only.

Soon after on a visit to London his friends were shocked by his appearance and sent him to the most famous doctor of the day – yes, it is the same Sir James Clark – who diagnosed nervous exhaustion with a threatening of phthisis, and recommended a winter on the Riviera. Sir James with all his Continental experience was still no further forward in the treatment of this disease. To Menton, Stevenson went and on the way home formed delightful friendships in the village of Barbizon where Jean François Millet had his studio. There he met an American girl, Fanny Degrift Osbourne. Stevenson returned to Edinburgh and announced to his horrified family that he had decided to go west – to California. This was the home of Mrs. Osbourne who was in the process of getting her divorce, and the next year R.L.S. married her and brought her home to meet his parents. Once again illness struck him down and he was advised to go to the high Swiss alps which had recently become fashionable for phthisis, and was recommended by Sir James Clark. There were more restless wanderings between Davos and the Scottish Highlands, with now and then a consultation with Sir James. Stevenson tried living on the Riviera, in Bournemouth, but eventually at the age of twenty-seven he decided that Europe held nothing more for him, and he quitted old Edinburgh for the last time. The first idea was to go to one of those hill stations in California much favoured by consumptives, but his wife could not endure the altitude of 6,000 feet and Stevenson decided to spend one winter under the care of Dr. Edward Livingstone Trudeau, at Saranac Lake, still a mountain village within 200 miles of New York. I have sat in the frame house at the end of the village where Stevenson wrote *The Master of Ballantrae*. His health improved a little under Dr. Trudeau, but presently the couple moved back to California, and the idea came up that a cruise among the South Sea Islands would be beneficial. Certainly Stevenson found it easier to breathe in soft moist airs. He hired a 95 foot schooner which sailed like a bird and had a luxurious saloon. The story of their voyages to Hawaii, Tahiti, and later to the Gilbert Islands and Samoa make the theme of Stevenson's most delightful book *Travel in the South Seas*. By 1891 he was famous all over the world and he decided that the perfect climate was in Samoa where he settled in a place called Vailima. Here he enjoyed three wonderful years in a comfortable house, in sight of the sea. The temperature was never below 85 degrees at noon, or below 70 in the darkness, the perfect environment for the chest patient. Not a bracing climate, for there was a long wet season, but there were neither malaria nor other tropical diseases. Here Stevenson wrote some of his most famous books and became a father-figure among the natives. He had only two or three slight haemorrhages and it seemed that his tuberculosis had been definitely arrested. He missed his friends in Europe and immersed himself in the life of the imagination. A short trip to Honolulu brought on an attack of pneumonia. Back in Samoa one morning after some hours of activity at his last book *The Weir of Hermiston* he suddenly collapsed and died (1894) within a few minutes, at the age of forty-four.

Stevenson's illness holds a second mystery and I have heard a famous American physician say that Dr. Trudeau had told him that he doubted whether R.L.S. ever had tuberculosis at all. Trudeau was a keen bacteriologist and it may have been that failing to find the TB in Stevenson's sputum made him reach this conclusion. But this can happen in many indisputable cases.

5

Throughout the 19th century we hear the same desperate plaintive cry from the consumptives, but the majority were quite unable to express their despair and it is only here and there that we meet with a genius who could put into words the essence of this struggle. Katherine Mansfield, a New Zealand girl, had achieved a marked literary success during and before the first world war. Of all English writers she gives something nearest the flavour of Chekhov. Then she developed tuberculosis, tried many cures and many doctors, and it was the essence of her temperament to fight strongly against anything orthodox – especially the sanatorium which was the only treatment with any hope of success. In 1922 she came under the influence of a mystic George Ivanovitch Gurdjieff, a Graeco-Russo-Armenian, who was educated in the same school as Stalin at Alexandropol in the Caucasus. After years of wandering through Asia he started the 'Institute for Harmonious Development of

Man' in a chateau at Fontainebleau. This man was a fanatic who taught his disciples to seek a real life for themselves, beginning with the personal question "Do I really exist?" His methods included Eastern Dervish dances and a fantastic discipline. Katherine Mansfield made her leap into the future – and as it turned out into death – under this man's influence. She was convinced that if she had gone on with her old existence she never would have written another line, for as Gurdjieff told her she was dying of 'poverty of life'. She began to enjoy living at Fontainebleau, working in the garden, picking flowers, lighting a fire and washing in ice-cold water early in the morning. Then up a small, steep staircase above the cow house in a little railed-off gallery, Gurdjieff made her go each day to lie and sleep. There was a theory that the smell of cows and the sound of milking would have a beneficial influence. During that winter she poured out pathetic and terrible passages to her husband, John Middleton Murry, the critic, and in the December of 1922 she wrote to him her last letter about his visit. She felt that illness had robbed her of the strength of will needed to make the necessary change in herself. Her husband arrived at the Gurdjieff Institute soon after Christmas. On January 13th she suddenly had an attack of coughing and a great gush of blood from her mouth. Katherine died at the age of 34. She had died before she had time to make the real transformation she felt was necessary in herself. Gurdjieff had not solved her problem. In his opinion, she had not reached the goal he set before his disciples. Katherine Mansfield had not developed a soul.

6

What was really wrong with these gifted people? Robert Louis Stevenson utters their heartfelt cry. "I lie awake troubled continually by a hacking, exhausting cough, and praying for sleep or morning, from the bottom of my little shaken body. I have written in bed and written out of it, written in haemorrhages, written in sickness, written torn by coughing. . . . the Powers have so ordained that my battle field should be this dingy inglorious one of the bed and the physic bottle." These great and articulate invalids were not the only ones who suffered from the pangs of consumption, but they were able to express what was beyond themselves, what was almost impersonal since it belonged to thousands of other patients.

We search for a psychology of consumptive patients, and try to answer the question whether the disease struck them because of their talent, or whether tuberculosis was the ultimate reason for their fame. It is hard to find any common factor among these innumerable invalids, but one feature was found in nearly all. Their restlessness. Their frantic pursuit of health through changes of place and climate and people. To have the power to breathe easily seems a basic human right, yet it was something these patients never had, and a bout of fever or haemorrhage would follow the slightest exertion. A passion for movement became the strongest power in in their lives. Even John Keats had to give way in the end. Sir James Clark encouraged it when he told R.L.S. "Find a warmer and better climate, seek for healing air in the Mediterranean, in the Engadine Valley, or Colorado." Anton Pavlovitch Chekhov (1860–1904) a doctor patient tried to conceal his haemorrhages even from himself and he constantly suggested himself into euphoria, pretending disease did not exist. His life too was dominated by a restless nomadic temperament. He haunted the railway between Moscow and the Black Sea, then back to Moscow and in the country. To Venice, to Paris and back again. He even journeyed 4,000 miles across Siberia to the furthest point of the Russian Empire, the convict settlement of Sakaline. He was gloomy and cheerful by turns, and neither his illness nor his wanderings seemed to make any difference to his output of wonderful writing. R.L.S. showed more stoical courage and good humoured self-indulgence than our other famous invalids, and once he had escaped from Edinburgh and the influence of his father, he could sail happily across the Pacific and settle in the remotest spot of the globe. This seemed to subdue this restlessness. It brought a serenity, a power to theorise about himself which lifts him above the average patient.

So the consumptive is really two persons, and if he is also an artist, the divine self is at war with the wretched fever ridden body. It is certain that the stresses of genius are powerful enough to undermine resistance. These people have so much to achieve in a brief time, and part of their restlessness is due to fear of the disease and knowledge of its fatal effects. Their moving to and fro, their transitions of place seem to have small effect on their gifts. Their private letters and conversations are full of complaints, but their works are calm and luminous. Play over a Chopin Ballade or watch Chekhov's *Seagull.* Chekhov had his first haemorrhage at the age of twenty-five and for the next fifteen years was hardly ever free from fever and malaise. His writings are full of humour and comedy and although there is a tremendous social protest that belongs to the years before the Russian Revolution, those writings contain no element of defeat. Katherine Mansfield for all the brutal mismanagement of her last few years knew well the pleasures and serenities of the world. Another great member of this College of Consumptives was D. H. Lawrence (1885–1930). He spent years trying to escape from his illness and himself, in Ceylon, in New Mexico, and he comes nearest to being the psychologist of tuberculosis. The illness was in one sense a handicap but also it was a stimulus, and in any case their spirit would not have allowed them any rest. We cannot picture Chekhov or Chopin on the verandah of a sanatorium going for regular X-rays and graduated exercise. These unusual people had the indiscipline of genius and were their own hardest taskmasters. Chekhov and John Keats were medically trained and they knew even better than the others the symptoms, and the probable shortness of their lives. But all TB patients felt this frenetic haste. The illness drove them on, forced them to turn out in 10 or 15 years the work of a lifetime. Their romantic appeal coming partly from that restless pursuit of air to breathe gave them a particularly evanescent quality.

Though their lives were emotional and disordered, the works of these great artists show no trace of the morbid. You will not find in the poetry of John Keats anything which suggests he was gradually dying. R.L.S. preached a lifelong sermon on courage and optimism.

The melancholy tone we find in Chekhov is balanced by robust humour and is the essence of the Slav temperament, and his reaction to the sad ferment of his own beloved country a decade before the Revolution. François Frédéric Chopin too, this dandy of the Salons composed his music to please aristocrats like Countess Delphine. There is exquisite sorrow, hectic abandon, wild romantic gloom – but no flavour of hypochondria. D. H. Lawrence, a great and sensitive writer, lived among his own major obsessions, but it is unlikely he would have written differently had he been free from tuberculosis. His 'difficult repentance' was a personal secret he carried from childhood.

These people were subject to the daily stresses of their own temperament and the consciousness they had to do work that was lonely and difficult. If the toxins of tuberculosis made any difference at all, it was through accelerating the time schedule and shortening the hours when they felt fit enough to work.

D. H. Lawrence expresses the conflict best.

HEALING

I am not a mechanism, an assembly of various sections.
And it is not because the mechanism is working wrongly, that I am
  ill.
I am ill because of wounds to the soul, to the deep emotional self
and the wounds to the soul take a long, long time, only time can
  help
and patience, and a certain difficult repentance
long, difficult repentance, realisation of life's mistake, and the
  freeing oneself
from the endless repetition of the mistake
which mankind at large has chosen to sanctify.

Chapter 3

The Microbe Emerges

THUS far, our story of consumption throughout the 19th century is mainly a collection of personal case histories which have in common one element – the impotence of doctors to accomplish anything really effective, or to point to the cause of this mysterious malady. The famous consumptives tell us all too clearly what effect this illness had upon its victims, and we can be sure that for everyone who has left behind an articulate record, there were thousands who went to their graves undocumented, unsung. But that is hard to accept, and we grope for some objective reality, a cause we can see and feel and touch, and which may be tested by reason. About the middle of the century the beginning was made of finding this, through one of those totally fresh ideas which come occasionally and which beat for decades against intellectual rigidity. The man who achieved this, who comes before Louis Pasteur, proved what those Italian peasants had guessed in their instinctive way, namely that consumption is a contagious illness. This was easy to imagine, but a French army doctor was now to submit the idea to objective proof.

He was Jean Antoine Villemin who graduated in medicine at Strasbourg just after the mid-point of the century, and rose in the professional service to become a *Professeur Agrégé* at the medical school of Val de Grace, Paris. Although he held an orthodox appointment, Villemin who was one of those gifted individualists who commission themselves for a particular task, who do not need to be told, but set themselves on fire with their own inspiration. If they are lucky they find the Holy Grail. Jean Antoine Villemin conceived the idea that consumption was infectious through an invisible agent which could be passed from man to man, from animal to animal. Remember, at this date germs had not been heard of. He put the idea in a sentence: "The phthisical patient is to his messmate what the glandered horse is to its yoke fellow." Consumption was an infectious disease of man just as glanders is to horses. Without equipment or 'research training' he began to work with a few guinea pigs and rabbits and in 1865 actually succeeded in passing the disease from a cow to a rabbit. We are not surprised to hear that Villemin's idea fell flat: no one had any faith in his rabbits and cows. At this particular point Louis Pasteur was teaching chemistry at the Ecole de Beaux Arts and was becoming interested in diseases of wine and silkworms but had not yet begun to work upon human disease. Pasteur was perhaps the only man in France who could have appreciated Jean Antoine Villemin. Yet their spheres lay apart, and Villemin went on quietly with his teaching and his research, and lived through the siege of Paris (1870). Seventeen years later Villemin could not help a certain bitterness towards Robert Koch whose discovery of the TB germ in 1882 proved that Villemin was correct. Consumption was truly an infectious disease.

Robert Koch was a very different type. He took his medical degree at the University of Gottingen and after serving in the Franco-Prussian war, was appointed as the humblest rank of district doctor (kreis-physicus) in Wollstein, a village of four thousand people. In his spare time Koch kept a small menagerie of pets and probed into that curse of the local farmers, the infectious disease called anthrax. His wife presented him with a microscope and Koch, by now familiar with Pasteur's discoveries in the germ field, managed to demonstrate the microbe of anthrax in the blood of infected animals, the germ itself having already been observed in pure culture by Pasteur. Koch found something more. An anthrax germ can actually create spores, inert forms of the microbe which keep alive for long periods and can cause havoc among flocks of sheep. Robert Koch showed off his anthrax work to professors in Breslau. It was the first scientifically verified account of the passage of a germ from one host to another. It made a great impression, and Koch moved up to be city physician, and presently to the Imperial Health Institute in Berlin (Kaiserliches Gesundheitsamt) where with an instinct for the really big problem he began to search in the sputum of consumptive patients to find that microbe which Villemin had divined, but never discovered. In 1882 Koch found it, and named it the *tubercle bacillus*. This name lasted half a century until in a revision of bacteriological nomenclature it was rechristened *mycobacterium tuberculosis*. Koch also invented a system of scientific logic which verified that not only was this germ the cause of consumption, but that it could be passed from person to person, animal to animal.

So the modern outlook on consumption began on that March day of 1882 when it was demonstrated that consumption was not hereditary, but infectious. It was the greatest sensation in the world of medicine during the last half of the 19th century. There has never been a greater technician in medical research than Robert Koch.

A microbe cannot be seen under the microscope until it is stained and coloured, and it was fortunate that another German, Paul Ehrlich, who was a virtuoso with the new dyes that were being discovered by the German chemical industry, was drawn towards bacteriology. Paul Ehrlich introduced the method of staining the tubercle bacillus which, although it was replaced by an improved variation, was really the beginning of the modern technique. Robert Koch went on to further discoveries including the germ of cholera. Ehrlich invented salvarsan a cure for syphilis and received the Nobel Prize.

2

The news of Robert Koch's discovery spread quickly over the world in medical journals and was a message of hope for every consumptive patient. Within two or three weeks it was reported in *The New York World*. It offered a new scope for progressive doctors. Hunting the TB germ in a patient's sputum became a craze. It happened that a young Scottish physician, Robert William Philip, who had graduated in Edinburgh in the very year of Koch's discovery (1882) was on his way to Vienna, then the centre of postgraduate medicine. Philip intended to specialise in gynaecology, and like many others he tried out the new stain, demonstrated the TB germ, and on that day he had an apocalyptic vision. Here was an immense new world. Philip dropped the idea of gynaecology and went back to Scotland intending to specialise in the treatment of consumption. He got a frosty reception from the older physicians when he mentioned his new idea. He was told that this subject was 'threadbare'. Philip realised that if he was to study the disease properly he must have his own headquarters, and in one of those tall, gloomy slum tenements of the old city, up a dark winding stairway, he opened what was called in the language of that day a 'dispensary'. The word was used originally to describe those centres where the poor obtained medicine without paying a fee, a bottle of medicine being then the main feature of all treatment. Young doctors like Philip who were beginning to acquire private practice gave their services free. Certainly he dispensed some medicines but became far more interested in the background of these patients. He examined their lungs, noting the movement of the chest as the lungs filled with air, he listened to the breath sounds with Laennec's stethoscope. Yet merely to examine them, and test their sputum, without the prospect of being able to do anything further seemed to him a barren exercise. He began to realise that Koch's discovery could be used for the benefit of the patients in an entirely new way. Philip made a street map of those slum tenements within a stone's throw of St. Giles' Cathedral, and marked each case of consumption with a red spot. It was only too obvious that the idea of Villemin and Koch was correct. One case produced another and there were small family epidemics of tuberculosis under his nose. Therefore he insisted on examining not only the actual TB patient, but other members of the family. He called it the 'march past' – the group of contacts around the patient who, if they had no symptoms now would certainly have them in six months' time. Here in 1887 Philip founded a branch of preventive medicine which today we call epidemiology – the study of how a disease spreads in a family or a community. Of course he did not use this word, but the idea was original and it was the first time that such a concept was introduced. Naturally, the chances of the patient developing consumption were much increased by over-crowding, dirt and poverty, yet in those west end houses of the rich where his other practice lay, Philip had the same shocking experience: parents infected children, small family epidemics broke out, and since the rooms were kept hermetically sealed for fear of draughts, the TB germ was able to spread easily. From this simple fact of germ infection Philip took up the cult of fresh air with religious fervour. Not only was it necessary to blow away the germs in a room and reduce the chances of direct infection, it was something more. The open air life was not only a preventive, it was a necessity for all men. He said rhetorically "When I speak of open air, I mean not the air of the mountain top, but the air that is outside every honest man's window."

Now he carried this idea further by opening a sanatorium near the city which was an annexe to his dispensary in the old town. Here he could isolate his consumptive patients and give them treatment and the benefit from rest and open air. Presently his dispensary set-up included a farm colony, where patients taken out of their slum conditions, could practise country pursuits with a chance of remaining free from the disease.

Robert Philip carried out his ideas in Edinburgh for twenty years before they made much impression outside. He was gratified to hear in a personal letter in 1907 from Sir William Broadbent who had sponsored that meeting in Marlborough House. "I must confess that I had not fully realised the importance of your work and, while I looked upon you as a pioneer in preventive medicine against consumption, I did not know that your efforts went back twenty years . . . another fact I had overlooked is that in connection with the Royal Victoria Hospital you have fifty beds for advanced cases. I attach the greatest importance to this as a preventive measure. . . ."

Chapter 4

The Sanatorium Idea

THROUGH the last quarter of the 19th century and the first quarter of the 20th the treatment of tuberculosis is dominated by the sanatorium idea. Its first effective statement came from one of those eccentrics who rebel against the sacred beliefs of their time. A village doctor George Bodington (1799–1882) who went his rounds on horseback from Sutton Coldfield, near Birmingham, actually wrote (1840) a short dissertation on 'The Treatment and Care of Pulmonary Consumption'. The spirit of place favoured Bodington, for in that same village a hundred years earlier another original, William Witherington had discovered digitalis, still our best heart medicine. Bodington's recommendations included "A pure atmosphere, freely demonstrated without fear." For him, to live in and breathe fully the open air was one essential remedy. Farmers, shepherds and ploughmen who live constantly in the open air rarely had consumption, whereas the inhabitants of towns were its principal victims. In our English climate the cold is never too severe for a consumptive patient, indeed the cooler the air which passes into the lungs the greater the benefit, and sharp, frosty days in the winter are the most favourable. There could not be a clearer statement of a therapeutic idea which began to influence medicine only after George Bodington's death. Actually he set up a nursing home where he carried out a rudimentary kind of sanatorium treatment, but of course his ideas were ridiculed, and no one thought of reading his essay on pulmonary consumption until after he had retired from practice and it was reproduced in a Journal of Public Health. He died in 1882 the year of Robert Koch's discovery, and it might have seemed that his fresh air theory had died with him. But good ideas do not die easily, they may germinate late and it so happened a German physician Hermann Brehmer had read Bodington's essay and presently tried it out in a small sanatorium at

Gobersdorf (1859). He carried the theory one stage further and recommended not only pure mountain air, but regular exercise, and others in the south west of Germany opened similar institutions. Great sanatorium physicians were Hermann Brehmer and Peter Dettweiler. The most internationally famous centre was the Nordrach-Kolonie in the Black Forest which under the well-known Dr. Walther became so popular that the word Nordrach came to be the trademark of a progressive institution for curing consumption, and Nordrachs were opened in various countries. Tuberculosis struck heavily at the Celtic population of the Scottish highlands and islands. A notable pioneer in the Sanatorium movement was the Hon. Margaret Fraser, sister of Lord Lovat, who set up the first Sanatorium at Invergarry and later became (as Mrs. Stirling of Keir) Chairman of the National Association in Scotland. She lived later in the house which Chopin had visited in 1842. Prophets of the Sanatorium idea in England were Dr. James Walker and Dr. Vere Pearson whose vigorous personalities were impressed on a large number of patients.

2

Another pioneer in the open air life was Edward Livingstone Trudeau (1848–1915) who had started to practise medicine in New York City in the 1860s. He developed a cough, was diagnosed as a hopeless consumptive and given one more year to live. Consumption could be exceedingly virulent and doctors did not hesitate to give that drastic prognosis since there was no hope of averting fate by any form of known treatment. Trudeau had the logical mind belonging to his French name: he accepted the verdict and reasoned that if he had in fact only twelve months longer to live he would spend that twelve months in a place he loved best – the Adirondack Mountains, two hundred miles north of the city. Those inaccessible forests had not changed very much since Fennimore Cooper's Indians lived there. Trudeau settled in a log cabin at a place called Saranac Lake where he amused himself in his favourite pursuits, shooting and fishing, and stayed there through the winter. Next spring he went to see his doctor in New York who was astonished that so frail an invalid as Trudeau had ever managed to pass one whole winter in that appalling isolation. He pronounced however that the disease was no worse, and back went Trudeau to Saranac Lake. Eventually he made it his permanent home and over the years gathered round him a group of fellow consumptives to whom he became physician and father-figure. Trudeau outlived the New York doctor who had pronounced him incurable, he even outlived his own son, and for thirty winters and thirty summers he built up in Saranac Lake a famous sanatorium. He taught that open air is a cure but with it is needed the patient's acquiescence, learning to live within his limitations, giving the body time to build up resistance. This was of course a revolutionary idea. Dr. Trudeau's consumptives lived in small wooden huts with room only for a bed and a table, they walked in the snow and followed a wide range of activities. This open air craze astonished Trudeau's generation but it gave good results. Robert Louis Stevenson was among the many patients who came to Saranac and though he was not cured by Trudeau he certainly gathered strength.

Meanwhile sanatoria were springing up all over Europe especially in the Black Forest and the high Engadine Valley of Switzerland. Special value was placed on pure, uncontaminated air, and the patients reclined throughout the day on open verandahs, covered with rugs. At some sanatoria hearty eating was encouraged to the point of stuffing with food: graduated walks under the pine trees were the rule, and before radio and television the patients cheated boredom with books and flirtations. In this emotional hothouse where everyone had the same symptoms to discuss, hopes and fears oscillated like the temperature, and every consultation, each X-ray or refill was a battle to be won or lost. The medical superintendent, himself often an ex-consumptive, had to use his full resources to persuade the patients to stay, and some of these men developed a dictator complex which may have had beneficial effect, since tuberculosis weakens the will to survive.

3

The best insight we have today into the sanatorium idea is in Thomas Mann's novel *Magic Mountain* (*Zauberberg*). This appeared in 1924 but the background and detail belong to the period before the first world war. The magic ambience which Thomas Mann describes so well is the mountain slope above the village of Davos-Platz in the Swiss Engadine 5,000 feet up. A correct young German, Hans Castorp, comes up to the sanatorium Berghof on a visit to his cousin, a young officer who is there under treatment. By chance, Castorp is found to have a bit of a chill, and under the influence of the place he buys a thermometer. Before long he too is diagnosed as a consumptive patient and takes a room next to his cousin. The sanatorium Berghof has an international flavour and Castorp undergoes a profound education through meeting numerous characters who have deserted the plains on account of tuberculosis. There is an atheistic Italian, a Garibaldian full of fire and rhetoric who disputes throughout the book with the young Jesuit who stands for authority, obedience and high intellectuality. Castorp falls in love – very much at a distance – with a pretty Slav girl who is also a patient, and who disappears from the sanatorium leaving him with a nostalgic sweetness, her pencil, and a tiny replica of her chest X-ray. Then the cousin officer dies of tuberculosis and Hans Castorp is very much alone. Towards the end of this long story his Slav girl re-appears – but in startingly changed circumstances. Now she has a companion, she is the mistress of a huge colonial Dutchman, Mynheer Peiter Peeperkorn, a preposterous and unforgettable character, and one of the great talkers in European literature. He dominates Castorp and observes he is in love with the girl. Then the old Dutchman commits suicide with a subtle Javanese poison and once again Castorp is alone. The girl disappears. In a duel proposed between the Italian and the Jesuit the latter uses the pistol on himself. Hans Castorp's intellectual explorations come to an end. We are now at the beginning of the world war and the impression is given that Castorp, now cured of his tuberculosis, is to go down to the plains once again and fight as a German soldier.

This fascinating book of 900 pages gives us the authentic sanatorium atmosphere at the point when X-ray diagnosis had just arrived and artificial pneumothorax was being talked of. The sanatorium was a centre of health but also of extreme boredom with despair never far away. These patients feel that life will be short and although they long to go back to the normal world they come to dread leaving the protective environment of mountain and pine forests. Others had an equally pitiable fate. Their tuberculosis indeed became cured but they themselves became fixed in an over-anxious neurosis of inactivity. They could not leave and tried every means to stay. Many were permanently disabled for a normal life, not by tuberculosis, but by its cure. It is hard now to recapture this atmosphere, or imagine the aloof dedication of that sanatorium life, in which the godlike physicians who built up their patients' lives were as much bound to the system as the invalids themselves.

4

The alpine cure for bone and joint tuberculosis was developed by Auguste Rollier (1874–1954) at Leysin in the upper Rhône valley. He went there first of all to treat his own wife, but presently developed pioneer methods that largely depended upon exposure of patients to the strong sunshine above the snows. It was amazing to see these children, in splints and plaster casts, with various types of joint tuberculosis, lying outside – their skins almost black with pigmentation. These children improved remarkably and Rollier started a factory clinic and open air school. Although Rollier's method was used particularly for bone and joint tuberculosis, he believed that it could be applied equally to the pulmonary form of the disease – provided it was properly controlled. Rollier's charm and persistence in remoulding these young lives made him a permanent place in medicine.

Chapter 5
Tenth Birthday

ON the tenth birthday of the National Tuberculosis Association many must have been surprised that it had managed to survive. It was nonetheless in that first decade that the seeds were sown of our method of tuberculosis control so admired by other countries. Some progress had been made towards realising the Prince's slogan "If preventable why not prevented?"

Public health in the modern sense was hardly born. In the middle of the previous century that tempestuous pioneer Sir Edwin Chadwick had set up a framework of local health authorities, but he moved too fast, and had been obliged to quit the public service. Chadwick had tried to bully people into being healthy, and his fate had been a warning to all reformers. The health authorities had not risen much above elementary sanitation, water supply, drainage, etc., and a haphazard control of epidemics. Now thanks to the propaganda drive efforts of a voluntary body the handling of tuberculosis (the most serious infective disease) was being forced upon public opinion. This first decade of the century is the birthtime of preventive medicine. The Association can claim credit for its public education, pressure upon Parliament and health authorities, and teaching the ABC of health. Yet there was always a strong opposition to anything that savoured of compulsion. Freedom was guaranteed, including the freedom to spread disease to others. In an age before mammoth newspaper circulation or other media of mass education, the Association worked energetically. It reported in 1913 "Knowledge is never national. That which is discovered today in one laboratory is known tomorrow in every other. The only international rivalry in knowledge is for the universal benefit. Statesmen find that they may more readily embody in Acts of Parliament the laws of hygiene when these have been broadly accepted by the intelligence of democracies. The National Association has been one of the reflecting mirrors of knowledge . . ." Splendid words! Yet newspapers considered disease as repellent to their readers and therefore outside their province. Tremendous inertia had to be broken down before the average person would face even the word 'consumption'. The Association started 'pilgrimage exhibitions' – a quaint title for a collection of diagrams, pictures and leaflets which was sent round the country in a horse vehicle. In ten years a million saw this exhibition and it was even sent to Australia. By modern standards it was a crude affair, but those who promoted it had faith in their message. Sometimes the attendance at local shows was very large, and the two ladies who travelled round with it – a Miss Perkins and a Miss Williams – (their connection with the movement cannot now be amplified) – did their work well. By the beginning of the first world war some 80,000 leaflets and handbooks had been sold. Mobile health education was continued by an interesting personality from Leeds, Mr. S. Jacob, MA, LL.D, a forcible and many-sided individual who had taken a degree at the University of Bonn. Some twenty-six branches had been established and were setting up dispensaries and sanatoria, but the Association insisted that "sanatorium treatment without aftercare loses much of its power for good and may even be a waste of public money". The Westmorland and Cumberland branch erected its institution on the slopes of Mt. Skiddaw. Most famous of all the sanatoria was the King Edward VII Sanatorium at Midhurst, largely paid for by the King's banker friend Sir Edward Cassell. It still flourishes vigorously. The City of Manchester secured twenty beds at the voluntary sanatorium in Delamere Forest, and the City of Newcastle twenty beds at Barrasford Sanatorium, Northumberland. Most of these institutions were in the country, partly from the fresh air motive and partly from fear of infection. Many were entirely self-supporting since they catered for the wealthier patients.

By the year 1914 the income of the National Association had risen to £7,000. Its conference had become an annual affair and the fifth (1913) was opened by the Prime Minister in person, Mr. H. H. Asquith. John Burns, president of the Local Government Board, opened the 'Tuberculosis Exhibition' in Whitechapel, London, which was visited by some 180,000 people. The Association now had six 'colonial' branches in the Cape Colony, Canada, Newfoundland, New South Wales, South Australia and Trinidad. The vice-presidents included Mr. Waldorf Astor (afterwards Lord Astor), Dr. Horton Smith Hartley (later to be Chairman), Dr. Dawson Williams (editor of the BMJ), Miss May Broadbent (daughter and biographer of the first Chairman), Sir William Osler, Regius Professor in Oxford. There was also Miss Edith McGaw whose name we shall meet often in this chronicle. By 1910 Miss Freda Stickland had become Assistant Secretary and remained a devoted executive almost until the second world war.

In these early propaganda efforts the word 'health' and also the word 'welfare' are used with fresh meaning. Previously, one's health had been regarded as an inborn secret between the individual and his doctor: some were born unhealthy just as others were born poor, and society could not do much to change these natural states of mankind. The Poor Law Report of 1908 by the efforts of Sydney and Beatrice Webb proved this fallacy. Health had now come to mean not a fixed condition but an objective to which the individual could strive, while the welfare of the huge impoverished majority, the submerged and forgotten 'poor', became a phenomenon to be studied and changed. These opinions did of course belong only to the few visionaries in the Association who were always proclaiming that poverty was often the result of severe ill health, and that preventing tuberculosis would contribute to social uplift.

2

In these early reports we come across the word 'notification'. What today seems an innocuous though important procedure was the centre of fierce controversy. The idea that a doctor should break the rule of professional secrecy, violate his Hippocratic oath by giving the health authority the name and address of a person suffering from infectious disease was abhorrent. Notification in smallpox or typhoid had been practised for ten or twenty years, but why should this apply to tuberculosis? There were actually a few doctors who were privately sceptical about the 'germ theory', and Lord Salisbury, the Prime Minister, pronounced himself as against 'compulsion'. Once more the sad example of Sir Edwin Chadwick kept back progress. However, the notification of TB was introduced on a voluntary basis and not until 1908 was it made compulsory 'among poor persons'. Compulsory notification was one of the first triumphs of the National Association (1913).

There were other small but significant advances. A deputation waited on the Chairman of the London and North Western Railway and anti-spitting cards were put up in waiting rooms (today spittoons have disappeared even from small country pubs, though cuspidors survive in America). The Association's published list of open-air sanatoria revealed the depressing fact that there were extremely few beds available. The Association's quarterly journal sold 4,000 of its first issue, and we are told that newspaper cuttings were being "systematically collected and pasted into books kept for the purpose". For the first time the Association had a permanent Secretary, Mr. G. Seymour Fort, and the turnover of £967. 0s. 0d., was reached in a year. Offices were taken in the West End of London, in Hanover Square. It was only after the first world war that the Association moved to the more academic ambience of Bloomsbury where it had quarters in the building of the British Medical Association and remains there now.

The voluntary movement began in many other countries, notably in the USA where the National Tuberculosis Association was formed in 1904. There was also an international body which introduced (1903) the double-barred red cross of Lorraine as a symbol of the antituberculosis movement throughout the world. This symbol is still in use although the crescent is used in Moslem countries sometimes in substitution in order to get away from the crusading background of the Lorraine cross which represented a Christian, anti-Moslem movement.

Funds for the TB campaign were gathered in through the ingenious invention of a Danish postal official – Einar Hollbøll, who set up a 'TB seal'. The idea was introduced into the USA in 1907 but only came to Britain in 1932 when the Christmas Seal Sale was launched by Captain Alistair Thom.

In Ireland an original antituberculosis campaign was mounted by the Marchioness of Aberdeen, wife of the Viceroy. Health propaganda was given through women's organisations and a travelling caravan. Peamount Sanatorium achieved under Dr. Alice Barry an honoured place in treatment.

Northern Ireland did not have its antituberculosis organisation until 1946 when a branch of the National Association was established in Belfast.

During the first world war the sanatorium idea became firmly established by the most unpopular man in England, David Lloyd George. His famous budget of 1910 heralded a shift in the economic balance of power, and his Health Insurance Act (1912) threw the doctors into fierce opposition. The idea of organised medicine under a State Scheme has today become familiar, but we get near the tempestuous atmosphere surrounding Lloyd George's measures when we think of the next medical revolution, thirty-six years later – the National Health Service (1948).

After 1912 an insured person was entitled to free treatment though at first only wage earners were included, and not wives and children. It was obvious that tuberculous patients needed far more than ordinary treatment. The Association urged that they were entitled to special consideration and Lloyd George with another flash of intuition promised they would all have 'sanatorium benefit' limited to three months. The experts knew of course that three months was quite inadequate, and as for the sanatoria they did not exist. Nonetheless the right to sanatorium benefit had been established, though it was an empty right, and the Government set up a special committee under Mr. Waldorf Astor. On this body Dr. R. W. Philip of Edinburgh was a member. Its two reports form the foundation of our modern antituberculosis scheme.

It certainly confirmed the right to sanatorium treatment but there was much more. The whole plan, even nomenclature, was taken over directly from Philip's scheme in Edinburgh, including novel terms like 'contact' and 'aftercare'. It was laid down that a dispensary was needed for every 200,000 people. There was a long list of provisions to diminish infection, improve housing and control milk. A research fund and a bureau of statistical information were recommended. It would take ten years before these recommendations could be implemented. But for the second war this scheme might well have brought down the tuberculosis mortality to the low point which in fact it reached only in the late 1960s.

One forcible pupil of Philip's, Dr. Halliday Gibson Sutherland, collected a remarkable series of essays describing in detail the Edinburgh scheme. This volume was presented personally to Mrs. Asquith, the wife of the Prime Minister, by Miss Edith McGaw. Dr. R. W. Philip received a Knighthood.

The personality of this remarkable man impressed itself so powerfully on the antituberculosis scheme that we can pause to look at the sources of his influence and those of the woman who was his Egeria.

Chapter 6

Sir Robert Philip leads his Crusade

NO man ever created so diligently the background for his life's work, the right style of living, the right atmosphere. The imposing house in Robert Adam's finest Edinburgh square, Georgian architecture at its most gracious, was his headquarters, and to visit him there was an unforgettable experience. In a room at the back Sir Robert sat at his Louis Quinze table, behind him a row of porcelain jars in which the old physicians kept their unguents, decoctions and leeches. The great man sat lively and benign, his moustache was close-cropped and a pearl nestled in the black stock necktie. One caught a glimpse of buttoned boots. His voice was a deep bassoon, and the eyes were large, grey as the North Sea, calmly appraising. I never stayed long at that table without a sense of being adroitly probed, and once he had attained his object by careful cross-examination the whole man changed. With a negligent air he would mutter something about a bite of lunch and presently lead the way up the staircase to a tiny room at the back. Like everything in the Philipian routine these intimate lunches had become perfectly organised: grapefruit, sprinkled with French vermouth, fish or Irish stew, Stilton cheese, a cucumber eaten like an apple, and a light Sauterne. The gastronomic symphony came to a full close with the coffee he made himself. After such a repast, the only proper ending was a Havana, and Sir Robert was very solicitous about its rounded end. On no account must it be pierced – to do so was an outrage. And when lunch was over, he would ceremoniously throw open the window.

Each morning he walked to his University lecture with steps long for so short-legged a man. On that large head he wore a large bowler set jauntily, and he carried gloves and a gold-headed cane like an 18th century physician. Smoking a cigar he walked through

Princes Street Gardens to the gloomy hall next to his clinic. To his students the Professor of Tuberculosis was very much a character, and many stories were told.

There was his famous allocution to final year students, delivered very slowly in a nasal, hieratic tone with reverent pomp like a religious incantation. "Some of your teachers may say to you . . . cultivate a bedside manner . . . That, however, is not my advice . . . When you go to your patient . . . be your natural self – laying aside – *all pomposity and affectation.*" Those young men applauded the contrast between this excellent precept and its portentous delivery. In his early days, open air was a new gospel. His patients were puzzled by his oracular statements but they were willing to follow his advice, and I think he was displeased with them for being ill. Today we may smile at this insistence upon fresh air, but fifty years ago a rational style of living had hardly begun.

On two fixed occasions he moved away from Charlotte Square, at Christmas to Cap Martin on the Riviera, and August at Pontresina, five thousand feet up.

As a committee Chairman, Philip practised the magic art which conceals art. With his spectacles well down his nose he would drone through the agenda casting a soporific spell. He liked the speeches of other people to be short, indeed silent acquiescence pleased him even better. Now and then those large grey eyes would fix upon some uncommunicative member of the committee who would then feel inspired to put into words an idea which Philip had previously placed in his mind with that object. The proceedings rolled on with mesmeric ease and in the end the Philipian policy had been carried unanimously. His secret was the single-mindedness of a man who exploited one idea throughout a lifetime. In later years Philip became a lonely man in Charlotte Square and his first wife died at the age of ninety. His attitude to life, based upon the French, was rooted in the power of reason, and in the non-logical, non-rational world of human nature he was out of his depth. I hear still the deep bassoon voice, I scent the cigar, the vermouth, the spirit lamp and the famous coffee . . . symbols of a kindly and sagacious man and a great medical statesman.

2

During these early years of the National Association we often come across the name of Edith McGaw. She was the motive force in the appeal for money in the 1930s, and the organiser of voluntary tuberculosis dispensaries throughout London. Each separate borough had such a clinic and they were gradually taken over by the health authority, only one remaining – that in Paddington – where Edith McGaw lived. It remained, under her control, a voluntary enterprise until the second world war. Edith McGaw was handsome, wealthy, energetic, a woman with a passion for social services. She was a child of the Edwardian age when in contrast to abundant wealth (like her own) there was 'primary poverty' – the inability of so many poor families to lift themselves above the lowest level of existence. One important cause of that poverty, as she never tired of pointing out, was tuberculosis. It needed such heroic people to emphasise – even exaggerate – this idea.

Edith McGaw was an admirer of Sir Robert Philip for over thirty years. The legend is that originally she came to him as a patient and thereafter until the day of his death, his work was the main motive of her life. With Lady Philip she spent holidays with him at Cap Martin and Pontresina.

Then just before the beginning of the second world war, his first wife died and Edith McGaw became the second Lady Philip. A year after their marriage, Sir Robert died just over eighty, and six weeks later Edith McGaw joined the man who had been her lifelong inspiration. The new Paddington clinic for which she had gathered money but never saw, is today in regular use and on the outside there is an inscription to their memory.

3

Until the 1920s the National Association had financed itself, on a hand to mouth basis through subscriptions, occasional bequests, etc., but the need for a stronger backing was now obvious. Through the energy of Miss Edith McGaw a strong appeal committee was formed (1926) under the Marchioness of Titchfield, a lady of great charm and energy who thus began a long period of work for the Association, completed when she became the Duchess of Portland. A professional appeal organiser, Mrs. Frank Braham, was engaged – then a novelty – and the appeal opened in a style now become stereotyped: a Lord Mayor's dinner in the Mansion House at which the principal speaker was the Prince of Wales, and three years of well organised effort.

The objects of this appeal were:

A. Educational work through lectures and demonstrations in what were called 'Caravan Tours'.
B. Setting up of Care Committees for the welfare of tuberculous families.
C. Grants towards workshops for TB patients.
D. A sanatorium colony.

The 'caravan' which was the basis of the educational experiment was really an ordinary Morris van which transported cinema apparatus and exhibitions and the doctor who gave lectures. In charge of this was Dr. William Brand (Tuberculosis Officer for Camberwell, London) who was assisted by three 'medical commissioners' Dr. James Holroyd, Dr. Sidney G. Peill and Dr. Harley Williams. By today's standards, this cinema propaganda was rather crude. A famous historic saga 'The Story of John Macneil' described the progress of a patient with his wife and family who went through the routine of the Edinburgh dispensary, passed on to the sanatorium, to the farm colony where he was seen growing flowers, rearing pigs and raising cabbages. The story ended with John Macneil in his new home cured and happy. Though full of laudable instruction this film was a little too good to be human. Soon the costumes of the wife and the nurse became out of fashion and raised loud hilarity. The fact is that health propaganda was in its infancy, and health education hardly born. 'The Story of John Macneil' is now in the National Film Archives.

These 'Caravan Tours' penetrated into parts of the country which had never heard of tuberculosis before except in its tragic and personal aspects. They reached places which had never before seen a cinema film. The apparatus was clumsy and cranked by hand. The procedure was to drive up to a village, locate the hall where the lecture would be given. The first problem was usually to find the key, and windows and skylights had to be blacked out on long summer evenings. Long rolls of dark cloth were used and the medical commissioner spent the afternoon up ladders pinning up temporary curtains. Another problem was electrical supply, for the caravans penetrated into many remote places. Then there was the Chairman – often an unwilling notability who did not in the least understand why such a lecture was necessary – and in many cases was strongly opposed, since he was convinced that this particular part of the country had never had a case of tuberculosis. Often in the afternoon there was a special show for schoolchildren, and these were excellent publicity agents. Sometimes these children wrote essays and a few quotations will give the naive flavour of these early beginnings.

> "The doctor told us how some people thought of sanatorium life as something very terrible. But now we learned that when we are told by a doctor to go and rest in a sanatorium for a certain time we should obey, for I see for myself the good it makes."
> "When the lecture came to an end I was very reluctant to leave such a lecture and I wished it was beginning rather than ending . . ."
> "It is the duty of each to see to these things as much as it is the duty of each to give his allegiance to the King, obey the laws and glorify God."

Looking back, I am astonished at our faith in the advice which was all we could offer, for there was no X-ray diagnosis, no artificial pneumothorax, and no drugs, while TB clinics were hard to find. These lectures owed their success to the opening of people's minds to a theme which was strongly repressed. Often, members of the audience fainted, and there were angry questions at the end. Occasionally the Chairman disappeared – either through shock or disappointment. One caravan penetrated the most difficult terrain in the British Isles, the extreme north of Scotland, including the Outer Hebrides, Orkney and Shetland. The cinema projector had to be transported over rocks and by boats from small harbours. In some localities the cinema was considered definitely sinful and some of the stricter Presbyterian believers would not attend. Yet during those years almost every county and centre in Scotland between Muckle Flugga in the north of Shetland to the Butt of Lewis and the Mull of Kintyre was visited. One later acquisition was a cinemotor van – a cumbersome affair from which a film could be shown in the open air in daylight. I remember vividly occasions at the Speakers' Corner at Marble Arch, London, where talks were given among political agitators, temperance lecturers and cranks of all kinds. Ours was not by any means the smallest audience.

In these caravan tours I was lucky in my faithful collaborator, Charles Neish Duncan. He would go ahead and prepare the hall elaborately setting up curtains and a backcloth, in the style of the music hall of the period. He was brought up in the days of the dioramas, the pantomime, and the Shakespeare company which moved from town to town. He had played in every part from Macbeth to a red-nosed comedian. In his handling, cinema films never broke and there were no awkward pauses or breakdowns. I see him still, a quiet, effective, arresting figure in a black hat and changing into a smart white jacket. Whatever happened the show must go on. Neish Duncan was certainly a pioneer in health education.

Chapter 7

The Physician and his Patient

THE National Association was largely concerned with setting up dispensaries and sanatoria, and the Health Insurance Act was the first occasion when a particular disease could be treated without cost to the patient. These twenty-five years form a period of organisation. These men had little doubt that their efforts were going to be successful. They believed with the powers of a religious faith that if rest and fresh air were offered to the patient, and good housing and good food to the population, tuberculosis would disappear. In the course of this story we shall see the faith of these pioneers becoming justified, but for the patient who took ill say in the year 1930, the outlook was not so secure. True, he would have had a better chance of going to a dispensary, and possibly to a sanatorium. He would always ask two questions: "Have I got it?" and "Can I be cured?". We can glance at the physicians' methods.

Sir Robert Philip would set his patient on a low, revolving stool and after taking a meticulous clinical history would commence the examination of the chest. He laid great emphasis upon the movements of breathing. Were the two sides of the chest expanding evenly and equally? He would feel the shoulder muscles, and with two fingers would go over the whole chest, using percussion invented by Leopold Auenbrugger (1722–1809). (This Viennese physician was a music lover and had a keen sense of hearing. Placing one finger flat on the patient's chest he would tap the middle joint with the finger of the other hand and would judge from the hardness or hollowness of the note given what was the condition of the lung underneath. A normal chest gives back a resonant vibration, whereas if there is fluid inside, or dense fibrous tissue or a cavity, the note is quite different.) The physician would then use the stethoscope, and to the end of his life Philip preferred the wooden tube which Laennec had invented a hundred and thirty years before.

Rene Theophile Hyacinthe Laennec, a Breton born in 1781, had done much more for chest medicine than invent his wooden instrument. He had the hardihood to compare the results of his clinical examination with what was found afterwards at post-mortem, and he related the physical signs with changes that had actually taken place. His first stethoscope was a roll of paper made up into a tube and his wooden instrument came only after some years of experiment. After several breakdowns in health Laennec left Paris for the last time in 1826 on an agonised journey to his native Brittany. In twenty years of professional life he had founded the whole pathology of chest disease and acquired a European reputation.

Through Laennec's instrument the doctor picked up the soft whistling of the air as it enters and leaves. A change of note was important, and there might be crepitations which indicated fluid. Philip would have taken the temperature, for a tuberculous patient usually has some fever especially in the latter part of the day. The sputum would be examined by the carbol-fuchsin stain.

Such were the methods which were available to the physician say in 1930. The older physicians had something which was probably more useful than any of the above-mentioned methods, a kind of intuitive knowledge. Today when we search for more precision in diagnosis we ought not to forget that these older physicians, in their own style, were often just as successful in answering the patient's first question – "Have I got tuberculosis?". There was a further clinical method which certainly extended their range – X-rays.

In 1896, a professor in the University of Wurzburg, Professor Conrad von Roentgen, discovered an electrical force which could filter through solid objects and throw a shadow on a photographic plate. His first experiment displayed his wife's left hand – and there were the bones of the fingers and the wedding ring. At first X-rays were used only in injuries in bones and joints, but by the 1920s daring radiologists began to photograph the lungs. The vertebrae and the ribs stood out clearly enough, but what the physician really wanted was to see the lungs themselves, soft tissues containing air. These early X-ray enthusiasts were hampered by the inadequacy of their apparatus – the low voltage and primitive photographic plates. Slowly these deficiencies were overcome and during the 1930s a good X-ray picture of the chest had become essential in diagnosing pulmonary tuberculosis, although the older clinicians continued to insist that their personal skills were just as accurate. A further development of X-ray technique was the method of 'screening'. The X-ray image is thrown not onto a photographic plate for permanent record, but is projected onto a sensitised screen which gives a living picture of the chest and heart. The diaphragm is seen moving, the lungs fill with air, the heart beats. The skilled observer can judge not only the lung texture but the movements and changing shape of the heart. In due course screening became an essential technique. He would see fibrous tissue which had replaced the normal lung, he would see cavities – round holes, large or small – which are the end result of the tuberculous process. And of course he would see areas where the lung had 'collapsed' owing to interference with a local part of the air supply. The method called spirometry which measures air-capacity of the lungs and its functional efficiency was coming into use.

So we can say that the physician in 1930 using all these methods would be able to give a more accurate diagnosis, and had a sounder basis to forecast the future. (Anton Chekhov or Katherine Mansfield would have had a better chance.) D. H. Lawrence had tuberculosis for several years and seems to have had nothing like what we should consider adequate treatment – even for the period. The patient's second question – "Can I be cured doctor?". How was this to be answered?

2

We wander down a side road, away from the main highway. In the desperate search for a cure. The physician of 1930, would have to take note of a substance called tuberculin which for many years exercised a delusive power. This tuberculin is the fluid which has developed in the flask of broth when a colony of TB germs has been grown there. Tuberculin is the purified extract of the TB toxins. There are ways of standardising tuberculin so that it can be measured like a drug, and nowadays it is produced in solid form in freeze-dried ampoules. Robert Koch was interested in tuberculin chiefly as a curative agent, to be used as a vaccine, in small increasingly graduated doses. In 1890 Robert Koch announced his tuberculin to the world and the world went mad. Here was the man who had discovered the cause, was now to provide a cure, and from all over Europe doctors begged to have a small phial of this wonder drug. It is said that Koch himself had been opposed to making tuberculin public until further experiments had been carried out, but that he was pressed by the German Government. The result was unfortunate for the many TB patients and also for Robert Koch's reputation. Tuberculin is by no means a cure even though some physicians acquired special skill in using it. The results in non-pulmonary tuberculosis were better. But as a cure for thousands of patients, tuberculin was a major disappointment.

3

Tuberculin however does have a practical application in diagnosis rather than treatment. It goes back to a discovery made in Vienna by Clemens von Pirquet (1874–1929). After postgraduate studies in Europe and America he had become professor of children's diseases in his own city. He reported what was called his 'cutaneous tuberculin test' in 1907. Some insignificant condition such as a sore throat or bronchitis might prove to be an early sign of tuberculosis and tuberculin would settle the matter. This von Pirquet test is simple and safe, and it impressed the scientific world by the message it gave – that tuberculosis in town dwellers is very widespread. But it by no means diagnoses active disease. A positive tuberculin test merely proves that at some time in the individual's life there has been an infection with TB, but on the question as to whether this is in any way serious, the tuberculin test tells us little. It demonstrates the phenomenon called 'allergy', that is an especial sensitivity to the TB toxins which has been produced in a person's system only by some infection with the disease, perhaps months or years ago. Today von Pirquet's method has been superseded by a more delicate test introduced by Professor Frederick Heaf and this is used all over the world as the principal tool of the epidemiologist. It informs him whether an individual or a group have been in contact with tuberculosis, and if so to what degree. On these observations he can base a preventive campaign. So that tuberculin, intended by Robert Koch to be a cure, has turned out to be chiefly a method of epidemiological research.

Other refinements had been added to the repertory of the chest physicians. There is the blood sedimentation test. Dilutions of the patient's blood are put up in tall glass tubes. At first the fluid is pink throughout the height of its tube, but gradually at the bottom end the red blood cells have become a sediment. There are important differences in the blood sedimentation rate of a tuberculous patient, although these changes are found in other diseases also.

Then improvements have been introduced into the X-ray examination of the chest. A harmless fluid (lipiodol) is allowed to flow inside the bronchus and eventually gravitates to the lower part of the lung. Since this fluid is opaque to X-rays it gives an unmistakable shadow and this is very useful in outlining a cavity in the lung. Another special type of X-ray is called tomography: this by shifting the X-ray tube can give a picture in any particular plane of the lung. There are many other refinements but it was not until the 1940s that an even greater range of examinations was required when the new drugs came in and revealed that some strains of the TB germ behave differently from others. The phenomenon called 'drug resistance' became another important obstacle. This will be discussed later.

The basic skills of the physician – observation, judgement, and comparative assessments – are still needed, but at every stage he has greater refinement of technique.

Chapter 8

Collapse Therapy

ONE of the strangest methods of treating any disease came into use during the first quarter of our century. It is called 'artificial pneumothorax, AP, or collapse therapy'. Until the new drugs for tuberculosis came in the 1940s it was the physician's mainstay. This method depends on a basic fact of lung physiology. Our lungs are soft, air-containing masses of tissue rather like delicately made rubber sponges. Through their exceedingly thin walls the oxygen passes into the blood and is conveyed to the heart and the rest of the body. The lungs move freely so that new air breathed in through the mouth and nose can be brought into intimate contact with a thin film of blood which absorbs the oxygen and gives back carbon dioxide. Fifteen times a minute the lungs expand and contract and they move freely inside the cage formed by our ribs. This free movement is possible because the outside of the lung is covered by a glistening membrane called the pleura. The *inside* of the chest is lined in the same way. Thus two surfaces – the outside of the lung and the inside of the chest – can glide smoothly upon one another, like the finger inside the glove. Between glove and finger there is indeed a space, although finger and glove are in contact and the finger can move easily. Normal breathing depends on the fact that the lungs move freely without obstruction. This 'pleural space' between the lung and the chest wall, corresponding to the space between finger and glove, is a semi-vacuum of negative air pressure and this helps to keep the lungs fully expanded, otherwise each time we breathe out, the soft lung tissue would collapse like a balloon.

It was known that if the outside of the chest is penetrated by the stab of a knife, air rushes into the pleural space and replaces a negative air pressure by its opposite, and the lung is pressed down against the centre of the chest. Instead of being a delicate air-containing organ, it becomes like a solid sponge from which all air has been squeezed out.

The idea behind artificial pneumothorax is to use this basic fact of lung physiology to 'collapse' the lung artificially. The lung is thus put out of action and disease in the tissues has time to heal.

The idea was first put forward by a Liverpool doctor James Carson (1772–1843) an Edinburgh graduate who practised as a surgeon and was highly respected. In 1837 he became a Fellow of the Royal Society for his observations on 'Elasticity of the Lungs'. He actually used our modern term 'collapse' of the lung with the object of placing a diseased part in a quiescent state, leaving little or no disturbance from the breathing which would be taken over wholly by the opposite lung. James Carson recommended this idea in the treatment of consumption. "In these cases in which the disease is placed in one of the lungs only, the remedy would appear to be simple, safe, and complete. Haemorrhage from one of the lungs, the frequent prelude of consumption, if not immediately fatal would certainly be stopped by the collapse of that lung. It has long been my opinion that if ever this disease (phthisis) is to be cured, and it is an event of which I am by no means disposed to despair, it must be accomplished by mechanical means, or by a surgical operation." Thus wrote James Carson in the year 1821.

Unfortunately in the days before anaesthesia and antiseptics, there was not much hope for so ambitious a surgical operation, and James Carson's ideas were not put into practice.

The credit of rediscovery belongs half a century later to Carlo Forlanini (1847–1918) a graduate of Pavia who became professor of pathology in Turin, later returning to be head of a clinic in Pavia. He was well known for his cultured personality. Only in 1882, forty years after James Carson's death, did Forlanini write a paper proposing lung collapse for tuberculosis. The method was to inject air into that pleural space, through a hollow needle. In this way the negative pressure of the space was converted to positive and the lung forced towards the centre of the chest. To measure the amount of air he injected Forlanini used an ingenious system of bottles containing fluid. It was not always necessary to collapse the whole of the lung: a portion could be subjected to the positive air pressure. Forlanini wrote many papers and established an international journal devoted to this particular method. It was only after the first world war that artificial pneumothorax became established in Britain.

By carefully adjusting in cubic centimetres the amount of air injected into the pleural space, the physician can secure a high degree of what is called 'selective collapse' and can even compress the area where the disease is active, leaving the healthy lung in its normal state. It became possible to cause the emptying of lung cavities. The process of squeezing the lung could be kept going for months, by judicious refilling of the pleural space with air at intervals according to the X-ray pictures. In many cases this AP method was certainly curative and was generally combined with sanatorium treatment. Inevitably as with every method there were disadvantages. Sometimes, delicate adhesions would form between the outer and inner pleural layers, and would pull out a section of the lung, thus defeating the object of the collapse. Surgeons became very dexterous at cutting these adhesions through a narrow illuminated tube, and out of the original procedure devised by Carlo Forlanini a whole branch of chest medicine and surgery developed.

Surgeons like Rudolph Brauer in Hamburg, and Christian Saugman in Copenhagen, developed an operation called thoracoplasty. The principle was to give the patient a permanent collapse by creating a scar on the outside of the affected lung. There were numerous variations in this procedure and through the 1920s and 1930s chest operations became bolder and more successful. Presently a further development occurred – the actual removal of badly diseased portions of the lung. These lung operations came in before the days of antibiotics. The surgeons had overcome their early fear of opening up the lung. Before the first world war the well-known German surgeon, Ferdinand Sauerbruch (afterwards notorious as Hitler's doctor) actually began to do his chest operations in a negative pressure operating theatre set up at great expense. However, this was found to be quite unnecessary. The dangers of operating inside the thoracic cavity had been greatly exaggerated, and today lung operations are performed freely. Their main value is for lung cancer.

Thus until the end of the 1930s the tuberculous patient who managed to get a place in a good sanatorium would almost certainly be given artificial pneumothorax. He would know that his cavity was being treated on expert mechanical principles and that there was a good chance that the lung thus given a period of complete quietude would heal itself and gradually expand.

Artificial pneumothorax was the first strong therapeutic hope in tuberculosis since the beginning of the century. The idea of James Carson a hundred years earlier was being fulfilled.

Chapter 9
Calmette's Tame Bacillus

THE word 'vaccination' goes back to before 1800, and was invented by Edward Jenner, the English country doctor who succeeded in protecting his patients against that universal scourge, smallpox. This vaccination idea is simple. Introduce into the system the germ of a harmless disease and you protect the person against a more serious condition. A mild attack of cowpox (vaccinia) renders the patient immune to smallpox. Jenner's idea spread all over the world. Vaccination against smallpox became compulsory in England and other countries. A hundred years after Jenner, vaccination against typhoid fever was introduced and its value confirmed during the South African war. Plague and diphtheria were to be prevented by variations of the Jennerian principles. We are now to see the idea of protective vaccination applied to tuberculosis.

The full benefit of Robert Koch's discovery in 1882 had been slow in coming. True, Philip introduced the idea into preventive medicine to protect the contacts in those slum tenements but no kind of vaccination was possible. Something more specific was needed to protect whole groups and populations.

The public likes cure but is not much interested in prevention. The thought of anticipating a disease by scientific methods arouses only tepid interest. However, in France, two pupils of Louis Pasteur were working at the most important idea in tuberculosis during the middle of the century. Albert Calmette (1863–1933) who had done medical work in the navy and in Indo-China on snake-bite and snake antitoxins, returned home and opened a Pasteur Institute in the City of Lille. He managed to finance this Institute through his chance discovery of a mushroom which had the power to convert starch into sugar and alcohol and which was commercially exploited by the distillers. A few years later Calmette set up the first antituberculosis clinic in France. But his main interest was always the TB germ itself.

It is not a delicate organism like the typhoid bacillus. The TB germ has a dense, waxy overcoat which makes it very resistant, and it grows with exceeding slowness. Calmette began to make cultures on slices of potato soaked in glycerine, but the process required weeks. Outside in the yard Calmette kept a menagerie of animals, mostly bovine, and before 1910 he made an important discovery. Through accident, or inspiration, Calmette found that adding to the glycerine potato culture a drop of sterile ox-bile caused the thick yellowish clumps of germs to become less tenacious. Ox-bile encouraged the colonies to separate out and it became possible to isolate individual germs. Any culture of tuberculosis germs is in fact a collection of numerous families or strains which all give slightly different reactions. Every few weeks the bacteriologist must 'sub-culture' his organisms – that is, transfer a clump of germs to a fresh potato medium on which a new family would be reared. Calmette engaged to help him a veterinarian from Limoges – Camille Guérin – and between them they went on with the laborious toil of transplanting their TB germs over thirteen consecutive years, a total of 231 sub-cultures. Even when the Germans occupied Lille during the first world war, that weekly sub-culturing was not interrupted. In the year 1921 a notable change was observed in the habits of the organism which had been growing for thirteen years. In modern jargon, this would be called a 'breakthrough' but it was far from dramatic. Calmette found that after 231 sub-cultures a completely new generation of TB germs had appeared and though it outwardly resembled its predecessors the new sub-species had a different effect when injected into a guinea pig. The original TB culture would kill off the guinea pig in sixty days, when given in incredibly small dilution. As we say, it was an exceedingly virulent germ. But the successor of that same organism in 1921 was harmless. Its virulence seemed to have disappeared. Although the guinea pig did develop a type of tuberculosis, this was not fatal and seemed to cause no disturbance. And this new organism which could not kill the animal could still provoke that animal's tissues to defensive reactions.

So thirteen years' work had evolved a new variety of the TB germ which outwardly resembled its ferocious ancestor but had lost all, or most of its sinister power. The jungle tiger had become a domestic cat. It occurred to Calmette that he could use this harmless species to vaccinate a human subject, and in due course that subject would behave as the guinea pig had done – it would develop a resistance to the virulent TB without suffering any harm. It would behave like a vaccine against smallpox or typhoid. However, the really tormenting doubt was whether at some future date the harmless TB culture could return to its primitive savagery as though the domestic cat would revert to the wildness of the tiger.

This quest for a vaccine against TB which began at Lille in 1908 was not complete until 1931 when Albert Calmette had satisfied himself that his new vaccine culture was harmless, and these findings were confirmed by the Academy of Medicine in Paris. Everything seemed ready for the vaccine to be exploited on a wide scale as a safe and effective preventive against tuberculosis. It was given the name BCG – *bacillus Calmette Guérin*.

In 1922 Dr. Weille-Hallé, a French physician, had administered BCG to children with good results yet notes of doubt began to creep in, especially from outside France. In New York Dr. S. Petroff found (1927) that a BCG culture is never entirely pure. In fact each BCG growth on that bile potato was not a single family but a group of families, and some of them, according to Petroff, were capable of reverting to the wild state. These American findings were totally rejected by Calmette who continued to insist that BCG is a fixed strain which cannot return to its original condition. Opposition from the Petroff school became as virulent as the germ colonies they claimed to have rediscovered. And since this period was that of the re-emergence of Germany, the controversy over BCG took an unpleasantly nationalistic character. France and French-speaking countries accepted BCG, the Germans and some Americans rejected it. England seemed neutral. There was Dr. A. Q. Wells of Oxford who discovered that wild voles or fieldmice suffered from a type of tuberculosis, and from this animal he produced a vole bacillus vaccine which had a certain resemblance to BCG.

The issue of the vaccination controversy trembled in uncertain balance when there came one of those appalling disasters which can extinguish a creative idea for the time being. In a children's hospital in Lubeck, North Germany (1930) BCG vaccine was administered to a large number of child patients, and seventy-three of the vaccinated children died from tuberculosis. The Reich Health Authorities held a searching enquiry, and proved beyond doubt that the BCG vaccine given to these unfortunate children had become accidentally contaminated by a virulent TB culture kept in the same laboratory at the same time. Some of those involved received prison sentences, but the episode was like a death sentence upon the vaccine *bacillus Calmette Guérin*. It suffered a temporary eclipse and for the subsequent years faith was lost except by Calmette and Guérin themselves. Disappointment had much to do with Calmette's own death in 1933.

The period of the 1930s which was so unfortunate for BCG, saw the temporary eclipse of another great medical discovery – penicillin. Between 1929 when it was first revealed by Alexander Fleming and the outbreak of the second world war penicillin was hardly heard of. It remained a frustrated therapeutic hope.

2

Albert Calmette had not wavered, he had kept the strain going for forty years and repeatedly proved that it remained harmless and could not revert. The idea spread among his pupils and the Paris Faculty, and all over France doctors were giving the vaccine a trial. In 1932 Calmette reported that two hundred and eighty physicians had used BCG in eighty different departments of France, and a total of 514 doctors' children had been vaccinated. Of these some 507 children survived in good health and in only four cases was there any doubt of their wellbeing. Calmette took heart from this simple observation. Doctors are keen observers and do not lightly make experiments on their own children. In addition to this

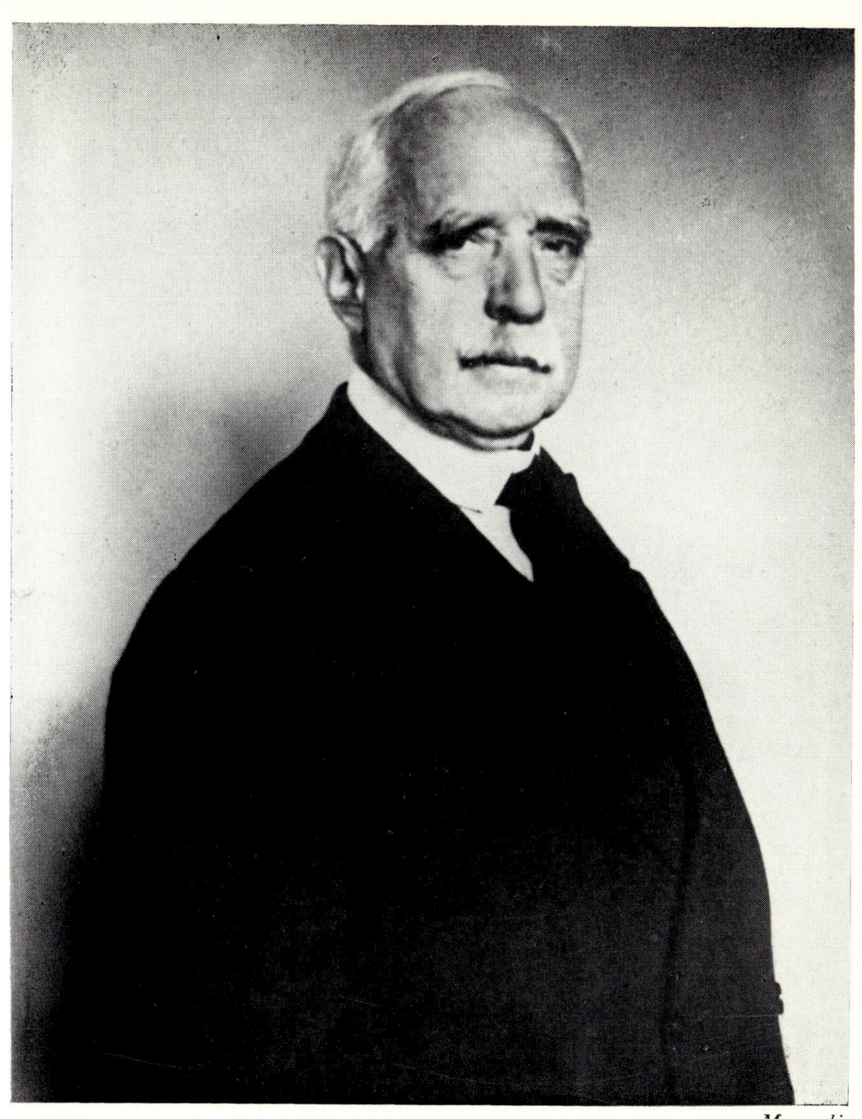

Maconochie

Sir Robert W. Philip

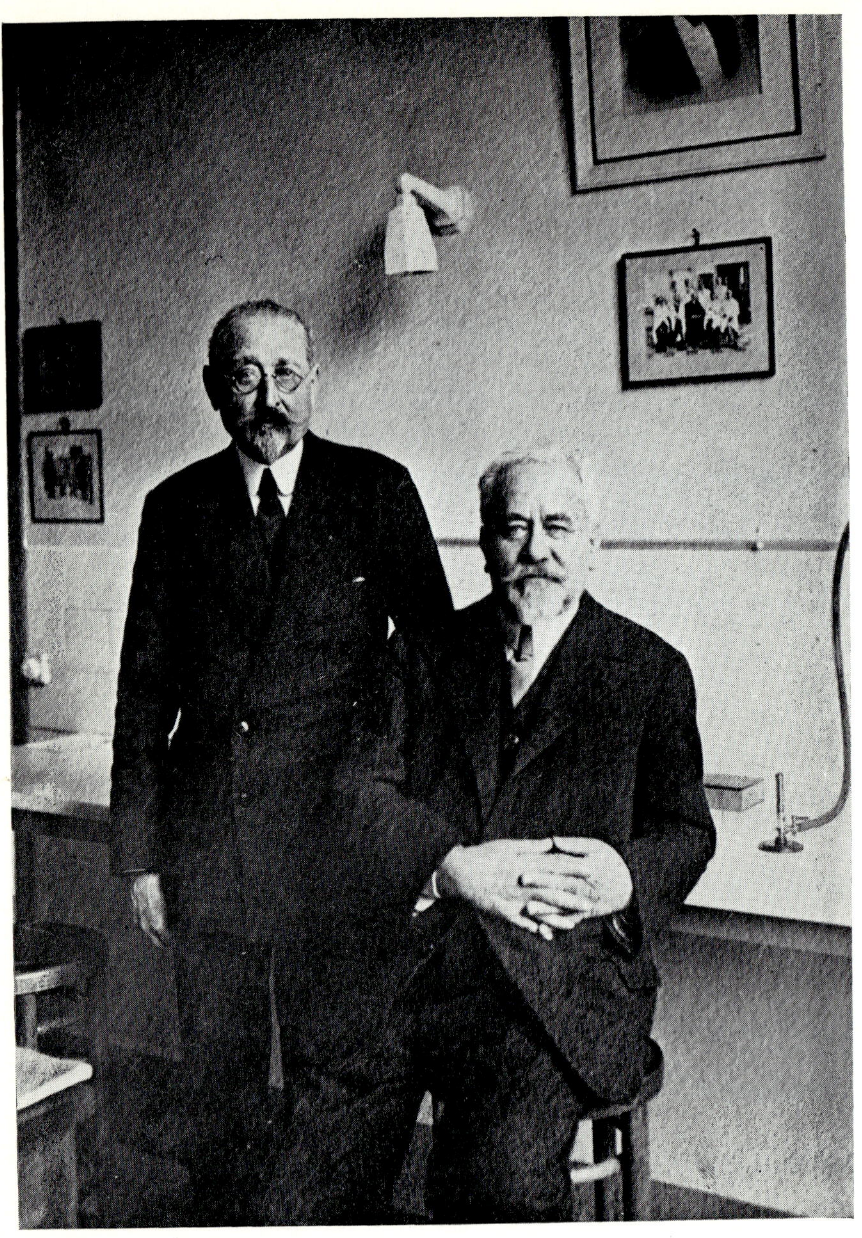

Albert Calmette (seated) and Camille Guérin

family test in France there were reports from outside the country which confirmed what Calmette had found. It became accepted in France that vaccination of newborn infants, especially where the parent is tuberculous, is an important step in preventive medicine, and a demand arose that all children – even from healthy families – should be vaccinated. Calmette's work was continued by his surviving partner, Camille Guérin, but the spearhead of the BCG vaccination campaign passed to the Scandinavian countries. Such great physicians as Arvid Walgren in Stockholm found evidence of successful protection by BCG and by the year 1948 some ten million individuals in the world had been BCG vaccinated. Camille Guérin outlived his senior partner by more than a quarter of a century. At the age of eighty-eight he worked on at the Pasteur Institute in Paris, a grand old man, cultured and vivacious, the last survivor of the great period of Louis Pasteur. With Albert Calmette there had been a perfect partnership and it is fitting that their two names should go into history as discoverers of the most reliable preventive method against tuberculosis so far revealed, apart from 'chemoprophylaxis' with drugs like Isoniazid.

In some countries BCG vaccination was coming to be widely used, while others e.g. the USA hardly employed it at all. Between these extremes Great Britain for long stood in a posture of tepid approval. With one hand we supported BCG, with the other we made gestures of cautious reservation. It was not until 1950 that the authorities decided to submit BCG to a careful statistical survey.

Under the British Medical Research Council, Dr. D'Arcy Hart undertook a strictly controlled survey of the vaccine, which included over 50,000 children. All these were schoolchildren, around fifteen years of age, who were first of all X-rayed and tested with tuberculin, and the negative reactors (over half) were divided at random into three groups. 13,000 received no vaccination at all. 14,000 were given BCG, and 6,700 the vole vaccine. A total of 56,000 subjects were re-examined three to five months later, then again once every fourteen months – with further chest X-rays and tuberculin test. The effect of BCG (or vole vaccination) was assessed and any complications were recorded. But no child was re-vaccinated. By

June 1955 every participant had been under observation between two and a half and four years.

What was discovered from this conscientious survey? It was found that of the *unvaccinated* children 1.94 per 1,000 did develop pulmonary tuberculosis, a proportion which represents what would have happened in the ordinary hazards of life. Those who were vaccinated came off very much better. Only 0.37 per 1,000 of the BCG vaccinated children (0.44 per 1,000 in the vole bacillus group) developed active disease – a reduction upon the first figure of unvaccinated children of thirty-five per cent. And among the *vaccinated* group there was no miliary tuberculosis or tuberculous meningitis, both serious catastrophes. These figures prove beyond question that around the age of fifteen, vaccination has a powerful influence in preventing adult tuberculosis. This MRC investigation had been well conceived, planned and executed. Doctors and nurses worked in the field, statisticians in the back room, with an expert committee presiding over all, under Dr. D'Arcy Hart himself. To keep 56,000 children under observation over four years in this conscientious style was one of the most ambitious projects ever undertaken, and the results are to the credit of British science. We were slow in accepting BCG, but at least we had proved its efficacy in a way that satisfied doctors all over the world.

There is one side-effect of a large enquiry like this which is worth mentioning since it has been observed in other such surveys. Any group of children, or adults, who are kept under observation by doctors, health visitors and social workers for a period seem to reach a higher level of general health, irrespective of whether they are vaccinated or receive any drug at all. The controls who were unvaccinated get this general benefit just as much as the vaccinated children, though of course they are not specifically protected against tuberculosis. Medical care seems to induce better hygiene and an improved psychological attitude. If proof were needed of the value of pure social medicine – quite apart from specific immunisation – here it is.

The MRC figures abundantly confirmed what Albert Calmette believed and what had been established in Scandinavia and elsewhere.

Was it worthwhile waiting to establish this knowledge beyond question, or should we have begun in England to vaccinate our adolescents ten years earlier? This is a hard question of medical policy. What one country invents, another develops, and a third confirms by statistics. The price of certitude is high, but so is the cost of preventable illness. Often figures prove what is already obvious, and leave unproved what is obscure. The British decision to go slow over BCG vaccination while this controlled investigation was in progress certainly does not prove that it is always wise to delay action until certainty has been reached. In the period when the method was out of favour the interest in BCG was kept alive in books and articles by a general practitioner, Dr. Kenneth Neville Irvine, who made this his hobby.

Calmette and Guérin had succeeded brilliantly. Their living vaccine sounds an alarm bell in the human tissues and if the real invasion with TB comes along, they are already prepared by vaccination.

Chapter 10
Manoel de Abreu

DURING the 1930s, the clinical physician had at his disposal fairly accurate methods of discovering – or excluding – tuberculosis in a patient who came to him, but this was an individual affair. He always hoped to get his patients in the early stage when treatment would be effective. Too often they came too late. The limitations of the purely clinical approach were becoming clear. Preventive medicine needed a method which could be applied to large numbers and would give a clue as to whether they needed more elaborate examinations. We needed to find the small needle in the vast haystack. The idea of what today is called 'screening' was still unknown, yet everywhere the tuberculosis physician was seeking a technique which would make his own work more productive, which would give him more patients in an earlier stage of the disease, and better results from artificial pneumothorax, surgery, or sanatorium treatment. It was hoped that the tuberculin test would have answered this need. But many adults give a positive reaction and this is by no means a sign of active tuberculosis, nor an indication for any form of treatment. A new method of 'case-finding' (the term was new) came from a totally unexpected direction, indeed as every new idea in medicine does.

During the first world war Manoel de Abreu, a young physician from Rio de Janeiro, came to study in the Paris Hospitals. He served in military ambulances, was decorated, and was for a time attached to the Hôpital Laennec in Paris. De Abreu was a man in whom the poet and scientist were close neighbours, and he conceived that it might be possible with an ordinary camera to photograph the chest X-ray on the luminous screen. He tried many times, but unfortunately the small opening he could allow his camera lens, and the weak luminosity of the X-ray tube, gave only a feeble result. In 1922 Manoel de Abreu returned to Brazil with his experiments inconclusive. Years passed before improved X-ray technology enabled him to get a clear photograph of the shadow on the luminous screen. Eventually he set up a frame holding a truncated pyramid of metal with the camera at its small end and the X-ray screen at the larger end. With this he photographed the chests of a large number of patients, and in 1936 demonstrated his results to the Medical Society of Rio de Janeiro. In 1937 he set up the first centre for what was called '35 millimetre fluography'. (The dimension refers to the width of the photographic film.) At a tuberculosis conference at Santiago de Chile (1935) he showed his invention to colleagues. By 1944 Brazil had more than two hundred survey centres for what had come to be called 'mass radiography'. No discovery in medicine is ever made at one source at one time, and it happened that a leading chest physician in South Africa, Dr. B. A. Dormer, invented this technique independently. But it was the prestige of de Abreu which enabled it to conquer the world.

Human subjects passed in front of the X-ray in large numbers since each photograph requires less than a minute. Then in a dark room these tiny pictures on a roll each about the size of two postage stamps were magnified and read by a skilled physician. Tuberculosis could be detected quickly, or at least a first suspicion would be aroused, and this would be followed by a standard size X-ray film. The real value of the method lay in what was done after the first photograph.

Mass radiography came to Britain in 1942 as a wartime measure, and twenty years later some three million miniature examinations were being made in a single year. The National Association took a leading part in popularising the method, and a departmental committee of the Ministry of Health which set up the mass radiography scheme met in its offices, with the Chairman of the Association, Sir Robert A. Young, presiding.

The first figures showed that nearly two per thousand of the general population had tuberculosis of such a degree as to require active treatment, while a further two per thousand needed supervision. Even before the end of the war, coverage of the whole country was confidently anticipated. The system was to regard the miniature X-ray film as a first rough screening only, and to advise those subjects who showed any abnormality to come back for a more complete examination. Lung cancer now began to emerge as a serious chest condition, though it was still overshadowed by tuberculosis. By 1948 some thirty-six mass radiography units were working throughout Britain. Only fifty or sixty in every thousand of those who came before the X-ray camera needed to be examined again with a large sized X-ray film, and of these only ten were found to have chest disease, and no more than four or five pulmonary tuberculosis. To detect this amount of disease was of course first-class preventive medicine and staff of these units earned full professional credit. As the method became adapted to peace time uses it was found more productive to confine it to particular groups of people such as pregnant women, and patients referred by the family doctor for a particular diagnosis.

Mass radiography was introduced into the Royal Air Force by Commodore R. R. Trail (1942) and developed in the Royal Navy by Captain W. D. D. Brooks (1944). In 1962 the Joint Tuberculosis Council declared that "Mass Radiography has been a powerful instrument in the attainment of the present improved position in regard to tuberculosis."

2

Manoel de Abreu returned to Brazil and made only rare visits to Europe. He was President of the International Union Against Tuberculosis when it met in Rio de Janiero. He was one of the most remarkable doctors of his day, dark, vivacious, loquacious. Large Latin eyes perpetually smiled in the olive complexion, and his eternal cigarette gave the impression of having remained alight since the previous day. He wrote poetry as well as philosophy, and in his late years devoted his leisure to mathematical calculations.

De Abreu believed he had found a method of using the force of gravitation as a source of energy. He dreamed that in due course this conversion would entirely replace nuclear and solar energy. He once showed me a photograph of a strange looking apparatus which seemed to consist of two pairs of horizontal bellows, and this was set up in a bathroom in his flat in Rio de Janiero. There was also a set of beautifully written mathematical diagrams which I was unable to comprehend. I do not know whether his theory would be adjudged sound by mathematicians, but if it should ever be realised, and those experiments in the Brazilian bathroom carried into the realm of practical technology, the name of Manoel de Abreu must surely be linked with Isaac Newton, and his mass radiography thought merely a by-product of unusual genius.

3

When mass radiography was used among special groups with a high incidence of tuberculosis, the tramps, those homeless wanderers in every city, were exposed to a new form of scrutiny. Their reaction shows how a new advance in preventive medicine meets with nearly insuperable human obstacles. Those who have children and fireside can be grateful, but there are some members of the human family to whom these things make no appeal. Their desire is not to go home, but to escape from home and all that home means. These are the Ishmaels, the wanderers, the beach combers, the nomads. They are incurably mobile, clinging to their ideal of personal freedom, a liberty purchased at heavy cost to themselves. One vocational enemy of the nomads is tuberculosis – the malady of stress and uncertainty. As persons, these nomads are as elusive as a mirage, but the type they belong to is permanent. A few pass off as conventional artisans, labourers, travellers, following normal jobs in this unusual way, but the majority are solitaries, seeking to preserve a lonely style of life.

In a large city there are organisations which cater for their peculiar needs, well-conducted establishments managed by the Salvation Army, the Councils and other bodies. Poor man's hotels offer – with a minimum of comfort – a sleeping place, and a place to cook the evening meal, conditions which represent the ground floor of social existence. Though there are few rules the clients (whose way of life is based on the assumption that any sort of restraint is unbearable) resent even what rules there have to be. Their chosen way of life is dearer to them than life itself. Yet compared to the park benches and church crypts where their predecessors passed the night thirty years earlier these modern resting places are sumptuous.

These nomads are mostly middle-aged men whom no woman has ever been able to hold or transform, and this is the time of life at which tuberculosis falls with special severity. The frequenters of these hostels are likely to reveal a high average of disease and because of their distaste for social conformity they are likely to infect others.

These men resent not merely the tiny acts of self-discipline which have to be observed by those who wish to be healthy, they loathe the slightest infringement on their private notion of freedom, especially the thought of tickets or cards that might lead to identification. Some of these ticklish individualists receive National Assistance payments, but they cannot be compelled to have themselves regularly examined. One lodging house invented a lure – a free bed for one night to the holder of the lucky number found in the queue for mass radiography examination. Other X-ray units found that the patience needed to wait even ten minutes in an X-ray queue was too great a tax upon these knights of freedom, and any hint of a return visit or clinical check-up was defeated by the disappearance of the elusive subject.

These rebels are prepared to accept the penalties of being lonely and dissocial – indeed to them this is no hardship. Why should not the world leave them alone? They never asked to be saved from themselves.

And what of society? These wanderers who suffer from tuberculosis in the ratio of nine or ten times more than other men in middle life are a standing pool of infection, indeed not a pool but a reservoir which leaks in all directions.

The welfare state has many mansions. This is more than a problem of hygiene and public health organisation. The nomadic temperament is found everywhere in all social groups.

Chapter 11

The TB Patient makes a New Life

THROUGHOUT those monotonous days lying out of doors on a sanatorium verandah, the patient would give himself up to daydreams, often dark coloured. Sometimes he suffered that temporary exultation of feeling, the so-called *spes phthisica* in which, having surrendered all sense of reality, he lived in the rosy world of the imagination. He was fit, he was healthy, he was free. More often, he was depressed and often sullen and aggressive to those who tried to help. He needed a leader, not only a skilled physician to cure his lung by collapse therapy, cutting adhesions, etc., etc., but a friend to help him towards a new life, and to plan the future more creatively than he could do alone. Tuberculosis can be considered a disease of personality, and certainly the patient's temperament plays a large part. Edward Livingstone Trudeau taught that the key to overcoming this illness was acquiescence: learn to live within one's limitations: make the best of what was available. Trudeau was a man who could teach this from practical example of thirty years in the Adirondack wilderness. The patient must learn, as Trudeau had done, to discover unknown potentialities in himself. He must teach himself not only a new life, but perhaps a new craft, or profession. Sanatorium doctors knew that the awful duration of the illness could gnaw away at hope. The patient needed a master and teacher, all successful cures were produced by the right physician in the right place. The TB patient had to contend, above everything else, with a malaise of will power, and although he would say – if only I could be free! – he encountered in himself some basic inadequacy of human response more deadly than the TB toxins. There is an innate indolence which compensates for its opposite – the restlessness. In a mysterious fashion the patient uses his illness either to heal or destroy himself. Successful re-ablement depends on personal inspiration and personal therapy.

Many sanatorium physicians were 'activists' who believed that the most important thing was to give the patient something to occupy his mind. This was the start of 'occupational therapy'. Patients took up some manual handicraft, basket weaving, woodwork or later what was called art therapy. Using a long period of sanatorium idleness to fill up gaps in the patient's previous education was excellent, and some sanatoria employed teachers of languages, shorthand, etc. All these things were meant to be constructive, but often the patient found in them nothing but illusion. "I learn to make a basket or do tapestry work . . . am I to go on with that kind of thing for the rest of my life?" One drawback of occupational therapy was its strictly temporary value, and for a patient with intellectual gifts the problem of the future was much tougher. His training fitted him for one thing only and that he might never be able to do again. In this group of patients there were many doctors who found their best rehabilitation to go on with this particular specialty to which they had been unwillingly condemned. Some medical superintendents lived in the sanatorium ever since that day a quarter of a century ago when they ceased being patients. They were not unduly overawed by the power of the micro-organism. "Look at me", they would say to the despondent individual in the bed. "I felt just as you do – but I managed to rehabilitate myself. You can do the same." The medical superintendent might go on to a few reminiscences. "In my early days we had no streptomycin and little pneumothorax, and I came to understand that beyond a certain point this disease is not to be taken too seriously. I learned to have a new objective in life, to become interested, forget myself and follow a big theme in medicine . . . the disease became insignificant. The same will happen to you." This was therapeutic rehabilitation at the personal level, but for a large number of patients something more systematic was needed.

2

In the early days of Philip's dispensary most of his patients came from the slums of the old City. With Philip, fresh air was a religious faith and he tried to take them away from their stark environment and give them a new chance closer to nature. Perhaps these patients had come into the City only a generation or so before. He set up a farm colony where from twenty-five to thirty men or women patients lived under a semi-sanatorium regime and were taught poultry feeding, harvesting and potato lifting. The farm colony idea was good so far as it went, and before 1914 it was a considerable advance on any kind of organised rehabilitation.

The question was answered against the background of industrial development following the first world war by a remarkable man, Dr. Pendrill Varrier-Jones. He began as a tuberculosis officer in rural Cambridge. Experience taught that patients who were advised to seek 'light work' were worse off than ever, for light work on a farm or anywhere else is hard to find, no employer welcomes the worker who has to go slow.

Then there was the inherent delicacy of the TB patient, the fragility of his resistance, and of course the danger, which his workmates greatly exaggerated, his power to spread infection. How was such a man to be trained for a new life and keep up his standard of living?

Pendrill Varrier-Jones was a man marked out by his appearance. His Arabic caste of features, the black curling hair, seemed to require the tarboosh of an Ottoman Turk, but he had Celtic fire and imagination and exercised a mesmeric effect upon patients. He could also wave the magic wand over rich industrialists. His famous industrial village at Papworth (near Cambridge) began with a squire's empty house around which wooden shelters were erected. When a carpenter to build these shelters was needed he was found among patients and the ex-TB carpenter became a permanent feature of the establishment. Small workshops were set up which grew in size and complexity, and slowly Varrier-Jones reached towards a village industry centred round a community of sub-standard workers – the TB patients. In an ordinary factory, one hundred per cent efficiency is demanded, yet Varrier-Jones was dealing with patients who not only began below this standard but whose working capacities could vary from week to week. Yet he still had the normal human being's desire to protect his family and be a member of a community. The capital of these men – their health and working time – was to be invested on their behalf in modern and efficient workshops. The patients began in the hospital, were promoted to the verandah, to the open-air shelter, and presently could work so many hours a day in the factory. Houses were built for those who wished to live there permanently. The original workshop grew into elaborately equipped industrial factories with machine tools, under professional management. Wooden furniture, leather goods, and printing became specialised and competitive trades. Twenty years after Papworth was opened the turnover from the industries reached the astonishing figure of a third of a million pounds.

Of course not every TB colonist relished the idea of spending the rest of his life in a community of fellow patients. Living in a cottage near one's work, being constantly under medical supervision, was not everyone's choice. On the other hand there were patients who felt a basic need for protective security symbolised by a doctor who knew their case, and a sanatorium near at hand to which they could retreat if necessary. During the 1930s the prestige of Papworth grew and it was imitated all over the world. Varrier-Jones was one of those natural leaders born to coax power out of a board of directors and money from shareholders, and he performed his art with a mixture of high idealism and worldly knowledge.

The British Legion Village at Preston Hall, thirty-two miles from London, opened in 1925 on a two hundred acre estate. Gradually it grew to have 450 beds and a hundred and twenty houses. Its carpenter's shop became a great industrial enterprise. Patients graduated from the sanatorium to the workshop and many settled in the village. Twenty years after the opening, some three million pounds worth of goods had been sold. The patients at Preston Hall were mostly ex-servicemen who became accustomed to living in the village, and a proof of the success of their lives there is that it was the rarest event for a new case of tuberculosis to arise in this community, although most of the adults were TB patients, lessons of prevention as well as cure being taught.

The success of Preston Hall was due to another remarkable personality, its Medical Director, Dr. James Boyd MacDougal. He was a benevolent autocrat but still an autocrat. In his younger days he had been an international footballer. More surprisingly he was a concert pianist. After he made a success of the Preston Hall Colony, MacDougal became impatient of gilding the lily through further improvements in a standardised scheme, and his organising skill and drive took him into a new career in the medical reconstruction of war-worn Europe.

The National Association itself had a colony originally started on the Edinburgh model but reconstituted in the 1930s. It catered for tuberculous boys who were trained in two simple courses: gardening or office work. The results were excellent. Young gardeners quickly found employment in the London parks and those who had chosen an office career were equally assured of work. Under Dr. A. H. MacPherson and Dr. William MacPhail this enterprise was supported by the Association until war conditions made it impossible.

A more sophisticated form of rehabilitation was 'art therapy'. This was developed by the artist Adrian Hill, who had himself been through tuberculosis at the King's Sanatorium, Midhurst. It was built up on a basic need for self-expression which many patients feel. Adrian Hill taught his patients to cultivate the 'innocent eye' which receives fresh impressions and transfers them to canvas. This filled up the monotony of the passing hours and enabled many patients to discover things about themselves. Inspired by Adrian Hill the National Association developed an art therapy scheme which provided teachers for a large number of sanatoria. A national competition was arranged and prizes awarded. Art therapy was an interesting counterpart to the more severe industrial forms of rehabilitation practised at Papworth and Preston Hall. In this type of rehabilitation and in many other constructive sides of social work Miss Nancy Overend took a leading part in the immediate post-war years.

Chapter 12

A False Summit

AS we draw near the second half of the 1930s we approach a summit. The mountain peak dreamed of by those ardent pioneers of the first two decades was clearly in sight, but not only in sight, it was now – or so it seems – within walking distance. We are reaching the zenith of that policy of tuberculosis control conceived before 1920, and thereafter the law of the land. Philip's dispensary scheme had been extended throughout the country, and the National Association had done its work well. The standard of treatment was higher than for any other chronic disease, and certainly than that given by any other country. True, the wealthy patient would go to Switzerland or the Black Forest, or to one of a dozen private sanatoria available in England or Scotland. But the patient who was not rich could nonetheless count on first-class treatment also. It came free of cost, and was in essence as good as in any private sanatorium.

Certainly there was one important defect in the system during those interwar years. Dispensaries and sanatoria were organised by the counties and county boroughs, and in the large and wealthy areas the standard was high. In the smaller counties the level was still inadequate. There were some sixty-one council and eighty-three county boroughs – large cities which had county powers. Over these the Ministry of Health exercised supervision, but British tradition is opposed to a centralising authority; everything was done by persuasion, and in some cases persuasion was not enough. Such was the British national tuberculosis scheme until the second world war put it under great strain, and Aneurin Bevan abolished it in 1948.

Many activities went on in the tuberculosis dispensaries in addition to X-raying and artificial pneumothorax. It was realised that the patient's home background was important. If he lived in an insanitary house he could get some help from the MOH and perhaps a new house and in the welfare areas a certain amount of assistance in food and clothing. A limited system of health care became available to tuberculous families through the Public Health Act, 1936. 'Special nourishment', thermometers, appliances and dressings, and the loan of beds and mattresses, payment of railway fares to and from institutions, training and resettlement in a tuberculosis colony, dental attention, wooden sleeping shelters, occasional payment of rent – besides a miscellaneous number of other encouragements for the patient and his family. These were administered under the tuberculosis officer and his female health visitors, and in many places there was also a voluntary TB care committee which in good areas might double the value of the benefits available. In addition to the tuberculosis officer these great physicians 'doctor air' and 'doctor nutrition' were frequently called in. At a point just before the second world war it could be said that the chances that a TB patient would get first-class treatment and rehabilitation were good, although in some areas they were greatly above the average.

2

The outstanding scheme among the county councils was undoubtedly that in Lancashire which was pioneered by another of those remarkable personalities this disease seems to produce. When the Lancashire County Council advertised for a central tuberculosis officer, Dr. George Lissant Cox was appointed. Such posts were unpopular in the medical profession, and it was said that Lissant Cox took the job to please his father, a Lancashire industrialist, who was a well-known Liberal party supporter of Lloyd George. This Lancashire scheme was unique in having its own tuberculosis committee and Dr. Lissant Cox gained everyone's confidence. He built up an elaborate scheme of dispensary areas each serving a quarter of a million people, each with specialist doctors and sanatorium facilities. There was a prestigious consulting staff, and an administrator of remarkable gifts, Horace F. Hughes. Of all this Lissant Cox was the inspirer and the master mind. His loud laugh was heard through the corridors of the Lancashire sanatoria, and his care was especially noted in the gardens, for he was a skilled fruit grower. Each sanatorium had its orchard and often the gardens were showpieces. He was undoubtedly the most successful director of tuberculosis work between the wars. When he retired he began a a new career in the marketing of Cox's Orange Pippins. The name was a coincidence but his success was remarkable.

Another very individual scheme was that in Wales which originated through the generosity of David Davies of Llandinam, the inheritor of a large fortune which his grandfather had made from the export of coal. This Welsh scheme covered two and a half million people in thirteen counties and twelve county boroughs, in a land mountainous and sparsely populated. The director was Professor Lyle Cummins who became professor of tuberculosis in Cardiff. When that other Welshman, Aneurin Bevan, abolished all county tuberculosis work in 1948 and set up his new model, no criticism was more bitter than that which came from his fellow Welshman who knew how successful the original scheme had been.

When mass radiography came in it was enthusiastically adopted in Wales and to set an example David Davies himself became the first subject to be examined. By a tragic irony he was found to have cancer of the lung and this became his last public appearance.

In this great development of tuberculosis from 1920 onwards the National Association had taken a leading part. Its conferences, held alternately in London and some provincial city, reflected the ideas of the tuberculous world. At the London conference in 1936 the 'significance of the examination of contacts' and 'the protection of the adolescent and young adults from tuberculosis' were the subjects of the first day. Then the conferences discussed closer co-operation between maternity and child welfare services, school medical services and the tuberculosis service. Tubercle-free herds in the years before pasteurisation of milk became universal was an interesting theme. At the 1937 conference in Bristol, propaganda

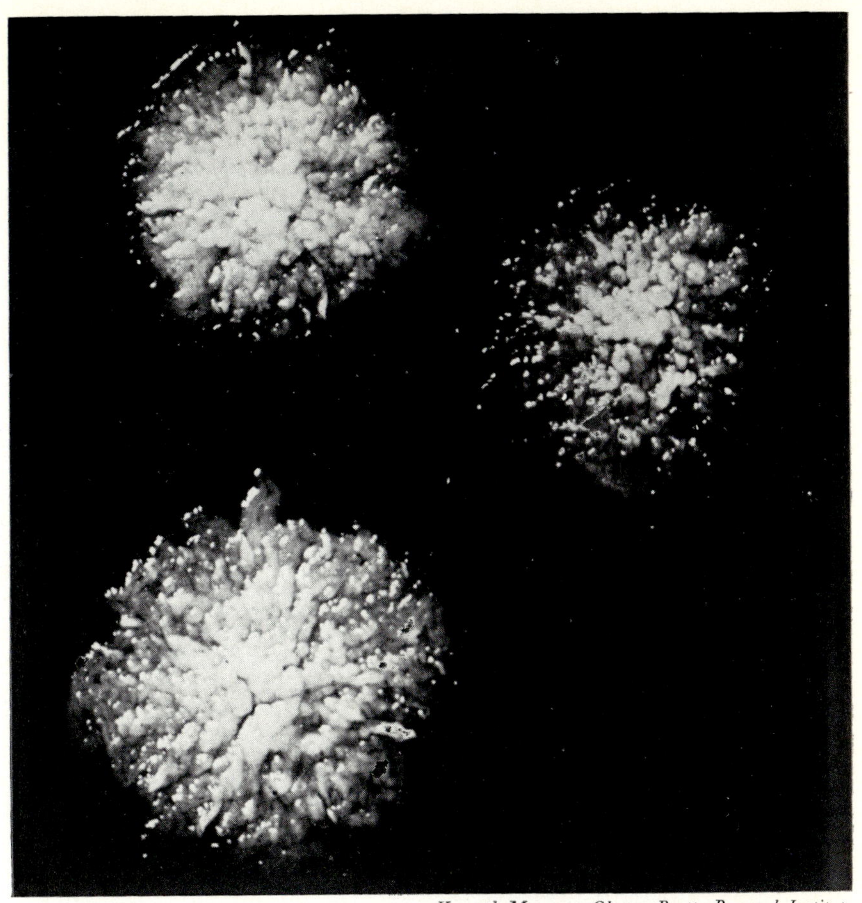

Kenneth Moreman, Chester Beatty Research Institute

Culture: Bacillus Calmette Guérin

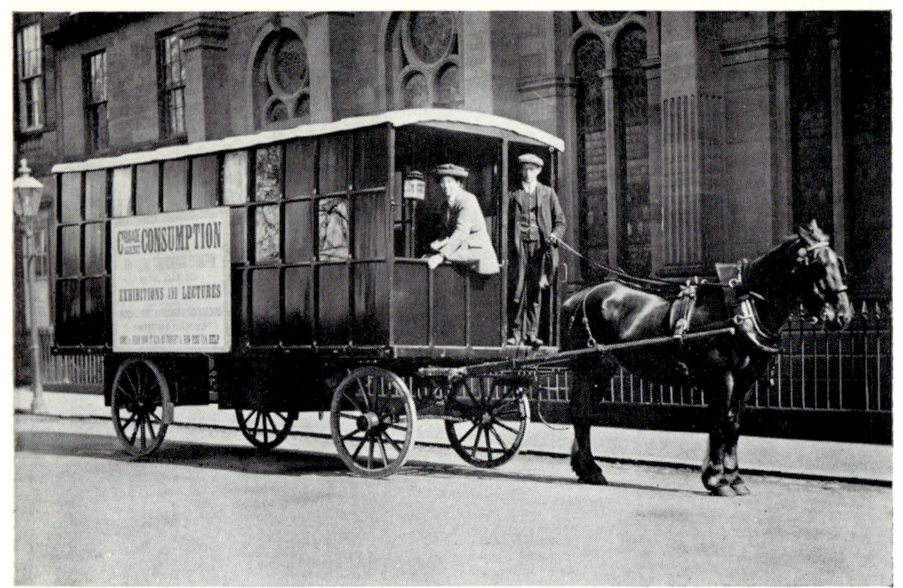

About 1912

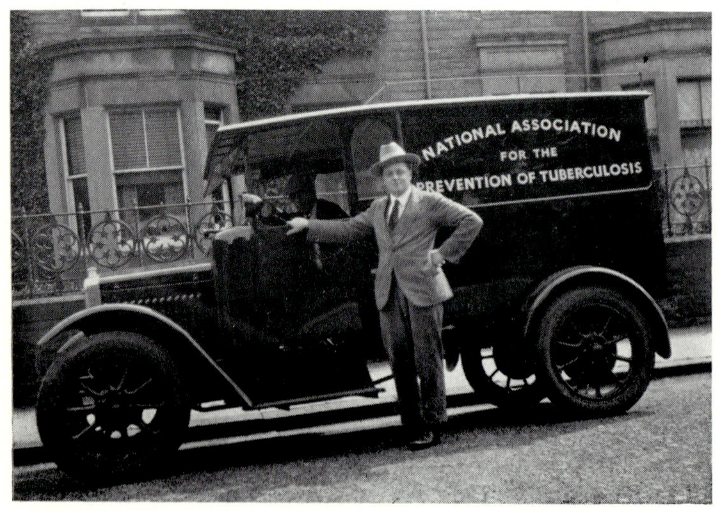

Around 1930

and publicity methods were discussed, as well as preventive institutions, especially open-air schools, and the equipment and activities of a tuberculosis dispensary. These conferences continued on their own unique plan: the doctors took their place on the platform with non-medical members, who represented the health authorities. This was an original feature of all the National Association did. It never permitted the subject of tuberculosis to become ultra-specialised, or followed only by those whose professional interest it was.

3

We have called this the mountain summit of antituberculosis work, and have compared these pioneers of the first two or three decades to ardent climbers who saw the mountain top clearly before them. A certain complacency was beginning to develop. There was a tendency to go over and over what had been achieved, to measure and remeasure the tuberculosis scheme as it existed. The country had come through the major depression of 1929–31, with its grim overtones of malnutrition, and there was a feeling that now progress towards normality was resumed – normality being the decline of the tuberculosis death rate to the base line. True, the ideals of the early pioneers had been to a large extent achieved; dispensaries, sanatoria, rehabilitation, social care, chest surgery were available to all, we have to remind ourselves that the only effective treatment of tuberculosis then available was the prolonged period of sanatorium residence, followed by dispensary supervision. These enthusiastic pioneers did not calculate that they were on the threshold not only of a world war – but a total revolution in treatment.

So although we have given to this chapter the heading of 'summit' it was a false mirage. The real summit was hidden by mists. In ten years more the prospects of a TB patient would be revolutionised from a direction which no one had foreseen.

Although Philip, the mouthpiece of prevention, did not allow for war in his calculations, his scheme of defence against tuberculosis was a rounded whole, and when war indeed came Britain was more fully prepared than other countries. The rise of the tuberculosis death rate during the first world war was prevented. This is proof that our anti TB scheme was effective. The new drugs could not help us, but they were among the earliest blessings of peace.

Chapter 13

The True Summit Emerges

THERE is a basic human instinct that the cure of disease must lie in herbs, flowers, roots, or in 'earths', that is mineral substances. For generations every type of remedy was used accompanied by the full resources of alchemy which was, in its way, a kind of science, and fully accepted by theologians and physicians. The doctor would not dream of prescribing belladonna, or stramonium or any other herb grown in his garden without first consulting his books of astrology which he used like logarithms. A patient's nativity, calculated on the date of his birth, forecasted his future destiny, and without this background knowledge the physician felt insecure. One great exemplar of this kind of medicine was Theophrastus von Hohenheim (1493–1541) usually called Paracelsus, and though skilled in the medieval lore of flowers and herbs, he did at last try to break out of the system and on one occasion publicly burned the books of the Greek physician, Claudius Galenus, usually called Galen, who had become accepted by the church, and whose statements about disease were received with the authority of scripture. The ancient Greek physicians certainly had faith in drugs, although these were comparatively simple, and they also knew that a drug could poison, indeed the word *pharmacon* meant both a curative drug and a dangerous poison.

Earlier in this story we have come across Paul Ehrlich who was the first to produce a reliable method of staining the TB germ. This was only at the beginning of his career, as the greatest exponent of the drug idea in the first part of this century. Ehrlich's method was to play with chemical compounds. He sat in a room overcrowded with piles of medical journals and scribbled his ideas with coloured

Footnote: Much of the material for this Chapter comes from "The Chemistry and Chemotherapy of Tuberculosis" by Esmond R. Long, MD, 1958.

chalks, his aim being to find that particular chemical dye which would fit the disease concept in his mind. He became interested in syphilis, a disease of which the organism had just been discovered, and after trying out six hundred separate combinations of arsenic, he discovered one, the six hundred and sixth called salvarsan. It turned out to be a cure for syphilis, and was man's first scientific use of an old alchemical idea. Salvarsan was presently replaced by less toxic drugs but the search went on for further compounds in which an organic chemical would be combined with a metallic molecule.

Robert Koch himself had observed (1890) that salts of gold were capable of destroying the TB germ, and at the beginning of the present century this idea was followed up. The theory was that metallic compounds of gold, mercury, or bismuth could exercise a catalytic influence upon the growth of the TB germ and bring about its destruction. A Danish physician Holger Møllgaard eventually built up a gold-containing drug called sanocrysin, which gave promising results in cattle and also with humans. The world of tuberculosis physicians felt a thrill of hope, but sanocrysin was much too toxic and in the end the results were disappointing. Gradually gold treatment went out of fashion.

In 1935 the German, Gerhard Domagk, discovered among the numerous dyes of the German *Farbenindustrie*, a substance called prontosil which he used with some success on human TB patients, although its value in other kinds of infection e.g. the streptococcus was very much greater. However, by the middle of the 1930s gold treatment had gone out and the sulphonamides (prontosil) also. At St. Mary's Hospital, London, there was a titanic figure, the bacteriologist Sir Almroth Wright who was outspokenly opposed to such methods – whether what was beginning to be called chemotherapy – or with the metals. In Wright's view the only possible cure for a bacteriological disease lay in a natural substance, something produced by the blood serum itself.

We have seen how, apart from pneumothorax and lung surgery, the treatment of tuberculosis was in the doldrums. The physician could only urge a drastic revaluation of the patient's life, and could not promise anything more than a very slow result at the most.

Alexander Fleming discovered penicillin in 1929, in that very laboratory at St. Mary's where Almroth Wright was supreme. Owing to the limitations of the biochemical technique then available, Fleming was unable to manufacture penicillin on a large scale. It grew in his flask of broth, extracts were undoubtedly curative, but gradually the essence – whatever it was – disappeared and there was no way of fixing it and making it widely available. Ten years were needed for this miracle to be accomplished.

In 1940 Howard Florey and Boris Chain discovered, through the technique of 'freeze-drying' then newly developed, a way of fixing the essential penicillin substance. What had been elusive and evanescent could now be preserved indefinitely. Penicillin became Britain's greatest gift to medicine.

Owing to the limitations of war time manufacture the British pharmaceutical industry lacked resources to manufacture the drug, and it passed without fee or licence to America where production was developed on a suitably large scale.

Penicillin, of course, was not used in tuberculosis but the idea that an antibiotic – a substance developed out of an earth mould – might have curative effects, set the scientific world afire. Those unhappy patients on long chairs on open verandahs had dreamed of a magic drug. One was now to be found which went beyond all that physicians had thought possible. Penicillin had been a tremendous exception to the then accepted rules of therapeutics.

Seven years after the last peace time NAPT Conference (1939) a way of curing tuberculosis was discovered which made all previous assumptions out of date. When the administrators were thinking of the year 1939 as the culmination of the dream which first came at the Marlborough House meeting, a scientist was working upon an idea, that same idea which had produced penicillin, but now with the extra confidence born of new techniques.

2

A Russian Jewish boy, Selman Abraham Waksman, arrived in the USA in 1910 at the age of twenty-two. He was born in a miserable village in the Ukraine, a mere collection of huts in a vast plain of black earth, and his early days were a frantic struggle to get what Jews value only second to their religion – an opportunity for education. In Czarist Russia this was hard to achieve, but Selman Waksman did have a certain success in the Latin school of his district and later in Odessa. When he failed in an examination upon a trivial point, his thoughts began to turn to the land where other Jews had found fortune, and he managed to get money to cross the Atlantic and after some misadventures found what was denied him in the old world. Selman Waksman enrolled at Rutgers (New Jersey) where he graduated in biology at twenty-seven. Here in this progressive college, the rest of Waksman's life was to be spent in a laboratory and experimental farm, and since Rutgers happened to be an active centre for agricultural research, Selman Waksman was drawn to the soil, or what Americans call dirt, and to those myriads of cellular living organisms which flourish there, especially families of microbes, fungi, and moulds. It was almost an uncharted field when Waksman began. An immense range of living bacteria goes on fermenting, breaking up clumps of earth, setting free its chemicals and as Waksman's knowledge grew, so did his field become even wider. He was to achieve success impossible in the old Russia. He went on with his search, examining peat bogs and that rich compound called 'humus'. He wrote papers, travelled to European conferences, even searched the depths of the ocean for bacteria. This whole world of nature, and the strange interrelation between the living soil and the living man became an immense though perplexing reality. A great international conference on the soil, was to meet in Germany in 1939, but never held. Then something he heard or read in a medical journal lead Selman Waksman intuitively to those substances that were now being called 'antibiotics'. This student of soil became a searcher for soil moulds which might be used in human medicine. If penicillin could be grown out of laboratory dust, then perhaps in his thousands of earth bacteria, there might be one which was potentially as useful. Waksman encountered many trials and many errors. In 1940 he produced a substance called actinomycin, but it was too toxic, and a later product clavacin was only a little less so. Fumigacin was less poisonous, but less active. Then in 1942 he made a big find – a substance called streptothricin could kill organisms which were immune to penicillin. Nonetheless, streptothricin was a little too toxic for human patients.

Among many outstanding investigators drawn to Rutgers by the prestige of Dr. Waksman was a young Frenchman, René Jules Dubos to whom (in 1924) was assigned the task of investigating the soil microbes which had the power to reduce plant fibres to humus. René Dubos went to the heart of the matter with what seemed a fantastic idea. Taking samples of the soil he noted which organisms were present, and in what numbers. He then 'fed' those soil patches with the germs of pneumonia and eventually prepared cultures which were tested against other pathogenic germs. This research culminated in the discovery of a new bacterial substance, gramicidin.

3

Alexander Fleming had made his great discovery through a process of intuition which lead to the unexpected. Being greatly drawn to one type of microbe – the staphylococcus – he made his experiments in that particular field, and the first success with penicillin was against the staphylococcus. Fleming appeared to stumble upon his discovery by accident, though this was not really so. The performance of genius is never accidental. However, we can notice that Selman Waksman made his discovery in a different way. He was actually seeking among those numerous soil organisms one that would be effective against the TB germ. He drew up his research protocol, assembled his assistants. His method reminds us of Paul Ehrlich's six hundred and six attempts to find salvarsan. Waksman isolated ten thousand soil microbes and carefully tested them. He found that nine thousand out of ten could be discarded, and eventually he narrowed his search down to 1,000 active cultures – the front runners in the race – and of these first thousand only one hundred were promising. These in turn were reduced to the final ten cultures which were tested with the most sophisticated methods then available. Of those final ten, the one which Waksman considered most promising was a mould called *streptomyces griseus*, and from this he extracted the essence which he called streptomycin. It is said that his son Byron Waksman encouraged his father to use streptomycin for tuberculosis, and in 1944 at the Mayo Clinic (Rochester, Minnesota) streptomycin was found to be exceedingly efficacious. In fact it was something like the wonder drug for which physicians and patients had been waiting sixty years.

The clinicians now took over the research and within the next five years some twelve hundred scientific articles appeared, and within eight years, six thousand. Streptomycin seemed to act in the human body by inhibiting the growth of TB germs, rather than by killing them, although streptomycin is not devoid of killing power. It is grown on a special medium of egg yolk and potato flour, and it has power upon other organisms as well as the TB germ, its potency even in tuberculosis varies according to the particular strain or family of the germ and one of the disadvantages of streptomycin is that there are some strains – called 'streptomycin-resistant' over which the drug seems to have no power. For the first five years streptomycin was used alone, but soon other agents came into use in treatment – neomycin, viomycin, cycloserine – but none of them seemed to have the unique power of streptomycin itself. Other types of drug, this time more chemotherapeutic than antibiotics, were being introduced. In Sweden Dr. J. Lehman discovered a fairly simple compound para-aminosalicyclic acid – generally called PAS. It has a powerful action though it tends to quit the actual tuberculous tissues where it is most required. PAS is generally used in combination with other drugs as part of a programme. Another pharmacological group under the name *isoniazid* was introduced in 1952 in America by three large pharmaceutical houses. It can be given by the mouth or injection. Isoniazid certainly arouses drug resistance in the TB organism, but this can be anticipated and avoided by a calculated regime.

4

Thus, nearly seventy years after Robert Koch found the TB germ it became possible to cure the disease by drugs, and an enormous revolution took place. Although a period in hospital is usually required at some stage it can be much shorter and the former insistence upon long rest and immobilisation disappeared. Tuberculosis was being conquered all over the world after 1950 and the only surviving obstacle – it seemed – appeared to be the high cost of the drugs and the clinical skill involved in administering them. Although the value of streptomycin was proved before the year 1945, another five years passed before it became available in Europe. To show how little was known of it during this period, just at the end of the war, I quote a saying of my friend Dr. John Lundquist (Director of the Swedish Tuberculosis Association) who said that the first time he ever heard the word streptomycin was not in a medical journal but from the lips of the King of Sweden, that omnivorous student of what is going on in the world.

Selman Waksman continued to work in his small third-floor laboratory at Rutgers, inundated with books and journals. He had donated to the University the manufacturing royalties obtained from streptomycin, and an Institute of Microbiology was built there. After the Russian revolution, Waksman had revisited his own village in the Ukraine and was depressed by what he saw. He had now become an American who had made the land of opportunity his own, and he knew that such success could never have come in the old Russia. He wrote a book *The Bible of Microbiology* which had a tremendous success and exhibited the hallmark of a good scientific work in becoming rapidly out of date. Selman Waksman knew, there is no end to change, no final point in what is called knowledge.

5

The use in medicine of these remarkable new drugs, many potentially toxic, demanded a new discipline. Apart from the assurances of their discoverers or manufacturers, there could be no guarantee that the drug would be safe or effective. All over the world physicians were losing their innocence about drugs, and were not so often inclined to follow the old adage – use a drug while it is new for its value is certain to decline! Then, the modern pharmaceutical manufacturer has to put enormous capital into his plant, and before he can invest time and money he must have some assurance that his product will be sold. One particular compound may cause harm to the human tissues. It is the ancient problem of the gardener – to find a weed killer that will not destroy the flower.

In this situation, the procedure of the 'therapeutic trial' was evolved. It is an exact and scrupulous way of scientifically proving the value, or otherwise, of any drug. First of all, the formula has to be considered safe on general principles, then it has to be tested out in sufficient instances to make the experiment scientifically valid, and statisticians require large numbers to work on. Then there have to be 'controls', comparable subjects presumed normal, or who are receiving a different drug, or no drug at all. In other words, the new drug had to be shown to perform something which would not have occurred spontaneously. These surveys require much time and the intellectual power of highly skilled physicians.

Great Britain has a century of tradition in medical statistics, mainly due to the pioneer work of Francis Galton, Karl Pearson and Major Greenwood. In 1953 our British Medical Research Council reported on the chemotherapy of tuberculosis, in particular on isoniazid in combination with streptomycin. Over three months some 364 patients were observed, a group which was divided into three sections. Some received isoniazid alone, some isoniazid plus streptomycin, some streptomycin plus PAS, and the effort was made to include in each group the same type of patients, so that acute and chronic disease was distributed evenly. Over three years the general condition of the patients improved and some gained as much as thirteen pounds. The temperature tended to come down and the sedimentation rates improved. The majority of patients in two of the three groups had now no TB organisms in their sputum. The general conclusion was that isoniazid plus streptomycin is a highly effective combination of drugs. It was further decided that none of the three drugs should be used alone, and for those who have already developed strains resistant to one of the pair – isoniazid or streptomycin – a change should be made in the treatment.

A great deal of the work of this highly expert survey was done by a remarkable physician Marc Daniels. Born in Cairo, educated in Manchester, medically trained in Paris, he was a cosmopolitan, a man who combined absolute intellectual objectivity with a winning personal charm. In early middle age he was struck down with cancer. He made a bargain with his unseen antagonist and decided to go on with his researches – at the time of his death he was in the middle of a BCG programme – as though nothing had happened, and when he was dying the bed was covered with papers dealing with the investigation. Some live many decades longer but do not achieve one tenth of what Marc Daniels accomplished in those last ten brilliant years.

Chapter 14

War Time and After

WHEN 1939 came, it was considered certain that tuberculosis would increase heavily in war-torn countries. This had been a lesson of history. Stress, malnutrition, the forcible migration of populations, these factors strongly favour the disease. It is gratifying to record that in Britain these grim prophecies were not realised. Our scheme for case finding and treatment measured up to the extra demands of war time, though in European countries the result was the opposite. In Britain, despite bombing and overcrowding, the closure of sanatoria or their diversion to wartime purposes, the rise in the tuberculosis death rate was not as great as had been feared. There were however several positive benefits which might not have come but for the war, or not so quickly. Mass miniature radiography was officially adopted and with it went a system of welfare allowances which heralded the Welfare State. The most important consequence was the realisation that there is a vast world outside Europe where tuberculosis could be accounted the most important disease in the Tropics. Neither BCG vaccination, nor the new curative drugs, came to Britain until after 1946. In the years 1940 and 1941 war time conditions did of course favour the spread of infection. Our swollen population suffered a violent mixture, and expectorating patients came in closer touch with non-infected individuals, and there was a severe shortage of houses. Long factory hours and the blackout were unfavourable factors, and the few sanatoria that remained for civilian use were inadequate and understaffed. By comparison with these grim years those urgent problems debated in 1937 and 1938 seemed to belong to comparative Utopia. At one point in the war 5,000 extra tuberculosis beds were needed and waiting lists were longer than they had been for thirty years. It was true, perhaps, that the pre-war tuberculosis scheme depended too much upon the sanatorium and too little upon home hygiene and dispensary care. The price of victory against this disease is perpetual vigilance. One important aspect of vigilance is a watchfulness against stereotyped ideas.

The transition from war time conditions to peace time recovery, called for great flexibility in the health 'establishment', and Britain was very fortunate that the Ministry of Health had, as its Chief Medical Officer, an outstanding man, Sir Wilson Jameson (1885–1962).

He had begun his career as a Medical Officer of Health, then became Dean of the London School of Hygiene and Tropical Medicine. He was moved to be Chief Medical Officer of the Colonial Office, and very soon succeeded Sir Arthur McNalty at the Ministry of Health. Wilson Jameson was an altogether unusual kind of Civil Servant. A man gifted with large imaginative intuition and flexible enough to look beyond current frustrations into a better order of things. During his period, the National Health Service came into being, and our post-war medical life of the country was greatly influenced by his ideas and his remarkable powers of persuasion.

The first problem of war time hygiene arose among the million and a quarter individuals – children and adults – who were evacuated from dangerous areas. True the absence of air attacks made sixty per cent of these people return to their homes later, but the intensive bombing which came in 1940 stimulated evacuation once again and about half the school population moved out to the country. Many hospitals were kept vacant for potential casualties. Food rationing made it hard to give the TB population extra protein and fat. Yet, notwithstanding great hardship, the general impression is that the first two years of war at least did not cause the serious damage to tuberculosis schemes as was expected. In the final year of the war (1944) the tuberculosis death rate was 58 per 100,000. This figure compared favourably with the corresponding statistic for the last year of peace – 60 per 100,000. However, there was no ground for complacency since between those two years the population had increased.

2

A world war and a global distress on a scale unprecedented certainly discouraged parochial ideas. In Britain we had come off better than was expected but the consequences in Europe were tragic. Dr. Marc Daniels who visited many European countries soon after peace, calls tuberculosis "the major health disaster of the second world war". It was the most widespread and most tenacious of all diseases in the festering communities left in the wake of modern war. Those who lived in Britain, Marc Daniels continued, saw the war as from outside the walls of a prison, and wondered what horrors would be revealed when the prison gates were opened. Those horrors were only too horrifying. The TB death rate in Warsaw, for instance, rose from 155 (per 100,000) to 500 in 1944. In Yugoslavia the figure rose from 95 to 263, in Vienna, from 109 to 257. Holland, in pre-war years, had boasted of reducing its TB death rate by one half in ten years: but in the war period it went up again by 134 per cent. In Germany itself the deaths do not seem to have risen so steeply and more beds were available in that country proportionately than in Britain, but after defeat the German situation deteriorated.

The organisation UNRRA (United Nations Relief and Rehabilitation Agency) was set up to send farm machinery, fertilisers, livestock, repair facilities and to eliminate actual starvation. Greece had suffered heavily and seeing that its pre-war tuberculosis organisation was primitive as compared with the standards of the West, the condition of the country was very grievous. What happens when a third of a million population had not a single TB institution or clinic? Dr. J. B. McDougal whom we know for his work at Preston Hall tuberculosis colony was sent to take this Greek situation in hand and set up mass radiography units. With supplies from the USA he managed to build up elements of a programme under great political difficulties in a period when one government would cancel the arrangements made by its predecessor. In Yugoslavia the situation was equally serious, and Poland was so devastated, its institutions so understaffed and under-equipped that it was like beginning again and the overworked doctors had to take on a complete reconstruction. Not least was the need for libraries of specialist books and journals.

3

To meet the severe shortage of beds the British Government arranged to send tuberculous patients to Switzerland where there was spare accommodation in the mountain sanatoria. Switzerland had always been the promised land for the TB patient, and even before the war a few British health authorities would pay part of the cost of Swiss treatment. Now, owing to pressure of public opinion, this idea of treatment in Switzerland was revived. Parties of British patients were escorted to Davos and Leysin where treatment was given under contract with the British Government. The Red Cross performed a useful service in guiding the patients from their homes, preparing them with clothes and looking after their welfare. The Ministry of Health had a medical officer at Davos who gave general oversight of the patients and a special railway coach was provided from Calais. On this train the French railway administration with a touching respect for the well-known tastes of the Englishman provided roast beef, something which the wartime English had come to think of almost as an unknown article of food.

Foreign travel is a matter of taste and also an art of its own. Many patients in Switzerland felt miserable without the British breakfast, afternoon tea or Burton beer, and they were irked by separation from families and the local cinemas. Being a successful patient is always a difficult vocation, and being a patient away from home has a special technique. This scheme came to an end as soon as there were sufficient sanatorium beds in England.

4

During the early part of the century the voluntary TB care committee became a recognised part of the scheme. It was an inheritance from Samaritan days, a realisation by the comfortable people who ran tuberculosis schemes that there was a disturbing gulf between man and man. The family of TB patients attending the dispensary were supported in various ways, by extra nutrition, or weekly sums for milk and groceries, the payment of domestic debts, and an occasional holiday for wife and children. These activities of course were entirely voluntary.

In 1943 mass radiography received official blessing as a method of case finding and it was realised that TB patients would not be persuaded to forsake their jobs and accept treatment unless there was some guarantee of security for the wife and family. It was no use saying to the patient – "You are an early case, you may not have symptoms now but your disease is likely to increase progressively. If you accept treatment there is a good chance of cure." This reasoning, though sound, did not go very far with the patient who weighed the immediate loss of earnings against the more vague possibility of becoming ill, and could not believe that a tiny X-ray picture could tell the doctor much. A new step in welfare was introduced under a Ministry of Health Memorandum bizarrely entitled 266/T. At first it applied to pulmonary tuberculosis only, because this was considered a disease which could threaten the war effort. Weekly payments were made from the TB dispensary. There had to be a hair line between such an allowance under 266/T and those from public assistance, and there were many local differences of assessment. One authority considered that marriage was a 'gainful occupation' and by giving the married state to go to a sanatorium, the patient was eligible for an allowance. A different authority considered that he was eligible only for an extra payment for domestic help. Patients could get weekly pocket money while in the sanatorium. This scheme despite its awkward title was certainly imaginative, and unlike anything that was ever known in this country before. The application of this complicated scheme owed much to one of the Senior Medical Officers in the Ministry of Health, Dr. Norman F. Smith. The Association had in most parts of England a voluntary care committee which supplemented payments under 266/T.

Mr. Ernest Brown, the Minister of Health (and a well-known pulpit orator), speaking to a national conference drew upon the scriptures quoting the deplorable behaviour of Sanballat, the Horonite, at a period in Hebrew history when workers were building a wall with one hand and grasping a weapon with the other. This character Sanballat went about mud-slinging and abusing the builders. It was encouraging, the Minister pointed out, that despite the malicious sabotage of Sanballat the wall of the city was in due course completed. He foretold that this would be the case with the new tuberculosis allowances. Under the Beveridge welfare scheme which came five years later welfare payments, which had been a novelty for the tuberculous patients alone, now became the norm for all illness. Once again workers in tuberculosis had proved pioneers in an important social change.

5

In December 1948 the National Association celebrated the 50th Anniversary of that day in Marlborough House when the few notabilities were suddenly made aware of the scope of its anti-tuberculosis work. Congratulations were received from King George VI, the Duchess of Kent, the Association's President, the Prime Minister, Minister of Health, and numerous Commonwealth statesmen and friends all over the world. These messages published in the Association's magazine make an impressive testimony to the international reputation it had acquired, especially in the latter half of the century. In 1898 there were thirty-six million people in England and Scotland, and seventy thousand lives were lost through tuberculosis. By 1948 the deaths were less than twenty-seven thousand, though the population had meanwhile risen to forty-eight million. This represented a saving of over a million and a half human lives.

The Association was turning its vision outside the British Isles. Even in 1948, The Rt. Hon. Creech Jones, then Colonial Secretary, put on record "I cannot speak too highly of the part it has played by its propaganda and educational campaigns and securing acceptance among Commonwealth peoples of the preventive approach to tuberculosis." Mr. Attlee, the Prime Minister, said "The NAPT has never lost sight of the human side of the tuberculosis problem . . . in this field especially there will always be a place for a voluntary organisation . . . ." It was thought that two pressing global tendencies would make an increase in tuberculosis almost automatic, unless vigorous measures were taken. Increase in population, decrease in food supplies. Every time a tree is cut down and not replaced, tropical storms wash away soil into the rivers, and scorched wastes cannot be converted back to arable fields. The study of the disease was not merely the actual local condition in the patient's lung, but rather a knowledge of a man's whole relationship with his surroundings. A new style of living would be required in this overpopulated and much abused physical planet.

In 1947 the Association inaugurated a series of large Commonwealth conferences which attracted members from all over the world. The later ones were held in the Royal Festival Hall, London's largest auditorium then newly opened. These owed much of their great success to the skill and energy of Hilda Walsh who joined the Association in that year and became Assistant Director in 1971.

The first post-war conference took place in London in 1947 in the Central Hall, Westminster, where the World Health Organization had been inaugurated only a few months before.
Mr. Aneurin Bevan, Minister of Health, electrified the audience by describing his new National Health Service, shortly to be born. It was not to be a centralised, state-run, soulless apparatus in which human personality would find no expression. Sanatoria and dispensaries would continue as independent, so far as possible, and the service would be carried out by boards and committees separate from the Ministry. Sanatorium treatment would come under the the new regional hospital boards but the individual aspects of the patient's life would remain with the local health authorities. The old Poor Law would be wound up, and welfare benefits would be higher

so as to lift the tuberculous patient above the need to appeal for Public Assistance. Local authorities would pay special heed to tuberculosis when allocating houses, and, the Minister believed, earlier diagnosis would make the TB death rate fall, and the existing dearth of nurses would not be prolonged. Of course the Minister's socialistic proposals came in for heavy criticism, mainly because they proposed to divide the tuberculosis service into two parts, so that the tuberculosis officer would serve two masters, the regional hospital board and the health authority. However it transpired that after the National Health Service was introduced, six thousand extra beds became available and the total of those waiting for admission came down from ten thousand to seven thousand. Months of waiting for a sanatorium bed became weeks or even days. But the problem of those who needed surgery – and at this period lung removal for tuberculosis was becoming popular – was as serious as before since the elaborate technique and after-care was required, demanding time and extra personnel.

This was the period when streptomycin became established as the best available treatment for pulmonary tuberculosis, and in 1951 a new agent (produced by Squibb, Hoffman Laroche and Bayer) came from Seaview Hospital, Staten Island, N.Y.; this was isoniazid which soon established itself.

6

The National Association was fortunate in having as its President, H.R.H. The Duchess of Kent, whose duties took her to Malaya where she took a special interest in tuberculosis. She found that in Singapore, eight per cent of the population were active cases. Some three years after liberation from the Japanese the Singapore Clinic was opened by voluntary subscription. In a short time it took five thousand patients per day, and was the largest in South-East Asia. Dr. G. H. Garlick, its Medical Director, was responsible. There was another equally splendid movement, the Lady Templer

Hospital in Kuala Lumpur, opened in 1952, and situated on a hill four miles from the city, at first with 140 beds in brick buildings. Eventually this would rise to 400 beds – all provided by voluntary contributions. In the Lady Templer Hospital several languages were heard – English, Malay, seven Chinese dialects and many Indian tongues. It was truly a multiracial institution and each State in the future Federation of Malaysia had its allotted quota of beds. The Lady Templer Hospital undertook chest surgery for Gurkha soldiers who were then on duty in the country. The idea of the sanatorium was the inspiration of Lady Templer, wife of the Commander in Chief.

Dr. George Herbert Garlick who directed the Singapore Clinic had held a number of medical posts in the territory. He was a resolute individualist whose dynamic viewpoint did not always conform to the stereotyped outlook of the administrator. For instance, he opposed the Government's case-finding programme, believing that in the absence of adequate treatment facilities, this could do harm. Dr. Garlick had sound reasons for every decision and no one ever questioned his personal integrity. He set off from Singapore to attend the NAPT Commonwealth Conference in 1952, and, alas, died suddenly on the journey. The Duchess of Kent spoke of him graciously at the Conference: "I had some personal knowledge of the tireless energy with which he tackled the tremendous problem of tuberculosis in Singapore. His loss will be most deeply felt not only by his colleagues at the fine clinic which he worked so hard to establish, but by many workers throughout the world."

7

Back in the 1930s we heard that the Marchioness of Titchfield persuaded the Prince of Wales to become President of the National Association, and raised a very large appeal fund. In due course when her husband succeeded to the Dukedom, she became better known as the Duchess of Portland, the very active leader of the

Association, no figurehead, not only leader and inspirer, but much more. Those who came to international conferences met a first-class Chairman of charm and authority. What was done so gracefully by her on the platform was no mere ceremonial attitude: it was the natural accomplishment. No one was more impatient with empty formality and red tape and her skill in public relations was an enormous asset. In 1958 the Duchess became a Dame Commander of the Order of the British Empire, a tribute to hard work and varied human gifts.

Not long before the Association was born, a young physician, Robert Arthur Young, qualified from the Middlesex Hospital. He wrote his examinations with a quill pen yet lived on to the age of scientific medicine, becoming the most famous chest consultant of his day. He first met with tuberculosis at a time when some doctors reluctantly accepted what they sceptically called 'the bacillary theory', when the physician had no X-rays, no effective drugs, no pneumothorax. Dr. Robert Young saw the rise and fall of curative tuberculin, the use and presently disuse of artificial pneumothorax, and the brief reign of gold treatment. He lived on into the promised land of mass radiography, antibiotics, and chest surgery. His reputation as a consulting physician began before the first world war and by the 1920s he had become unassailable, though he was not knighted until 1947. He was the leader of the team of chest specialists whose efforts helped to prolong the life of King George VI. For more than fifteen years after he retired from hospital in 1936, Sir Robert was as busy as ever as a consultant. Meanwhile he had embarked on a new career. He succeeded Sir Percival Horton-Smith Hartley as vice-chairman of the National Association, and Chairman of the Standing Advisory Committee on Tuberculosis. RA (his nickname) was a masterly presiding officer, expert in the formula which unites opinion round the table. His long, wide head, the rich judicial voice, sparing gestures, all expressed authority which was unquestionably accepted. In his early professional life there had been rivals, but now he had only friends.

As a clinician Sir Robert Young was admittedly marvellous. He toiled at each case until he had exhausted every possibility of diagnosis and treatment. He took no short cuts but would ponder each symptom and there was never a risk that he would overlook anything. Sir Robert would put the X-ray film under his desk blotter, not referring to it until he had found out everything possible from eyes, fingers and stethoscope. By the end of the consultation every aspect of the illness had received scrutiny of a fine mind, though the patient was apt to be a little overawed. A man so steeped in Edwardian background might have found new ideas hard to assimilate, but his mind grew more flexible. He quietly assimilated radiology, antibiotics, and chest surgery, without giving up any of his more personal methods. Then, he was unbelievably gentle, and taught that gentleness is one of the most important medical arts. In the patient's interest he could be adamant. No question of administration or research was ever allowed to come between him and that intimate understanding of the sick person. His career shows how a great doctor could be produced by a form of purely clinical specialisation which is now almost outmoded.

Sir Robert Young was succeeded by Dr. Norman Lloyd Rusby, physician to the London Hospital and Victoria Park Chest Hospital, and a leading specialist in diseases of the chest.

Chapter 15

Tuberculosis in the Tropics

COMPARE two slides under the microscope. Each shows clumps of red-stained rods – micro-organisms – and the two slides appear to be absolutely identical. Yet they show completely different organisms, which cause entirely different diseases. The first is our old acquaintance the tubercle bacillus (mycobacterium tuberculosis), the other is the microbe of that ancient curse leprosy. Outwardly, on a microscopic slide, the two microbes look the same, but their effects are very different. Only when we try to culture them does any difference appear. The leprosy bacillus has resisted attempts to grow it artificially. Today leprosy is being controlled in the tropics just as it has been eliminated from Britain. In India it is becoming rare for a physician to meet with a case. Yet tuberculosis is still undefeated. Leprosy was common in Old Testament times, and tuberculosis has certainly been identified in a skeleton of one of the Pharaohs going back to 1500 BC. We may conjecture that at some remote point in pre-history two strains of the one organism separated, evolved different habits and attacked human beings in different ways. This kind of thing happens with all living organisms, they are subject to mutations, alterations in habits and growth. In this case, both branches of the family have remained virulent, and these two infections – leprosy and tuberculosis – have scourged mankind for longer than any other evil known to history. Throughout the middle ages leprosy was common all over Europe and we have heard of the leper wearing a white robe and ringing his bell, shunned by the community. It was Dr. Armauer Hansen, a physician of Bergen, Norway, who exploded the theory that leprosy is hereditary, when he showed this *Lepra* bacillus under the microscope, nearly ten years before Robert Koch found the TB organism.

At the end of the second world war tuberculosis was the most important disease in the tropics. Malaria was being controlled with DDT and drugs: trypanosomiasis conquered by control of the tsetse fly and animal carriers: yellow fever virtually eliminated from tropical cities through rigid mosquito hygiene: leprosy becoming rarer . . . yet tuberculosis still remains an important 'tropical' disease which requires all the perseverance of public health experts.

Racial inheritance does mean something in one's liability to develop tuberculosis. Even in 1884 Robert Koch demonstrated that fieldmice infected with TB germs were more likely to succumb than white mice, and throughout the world human races vary, especially in the New World and the tropics. We quote from an American author:

> "In the great American city, the health inheritance is far from being uniform; it is patchy in the extreme; it is, indeed, a crazy quilt with each race representing a square in the design. As regards the colour tones of this imaginary quilt, it can be conceived in a general way that the squares dyed in striking or violent colours represent the primitive race elements or, in other words, the highly susceptible race components. We may imagine for instance, the square of the quilt labelled Mexican to be startling red; that the square labelled Indian to be a flaming purple; that the square labelled Negro is more subdued purple, and that the square labelled Puerto Rican is a vivid pink. Still using the colour simile to clarify our idea, we believe that the crazy quilt idea is not identical in any two great American cities. The Mexican square is more startling red in Los Angeles than in Chicago, a more flaming red in Chicago than in New York. The Negro square is more strikingly purple in Chicago than in Los Angeles, and the Puerto Rican pink is more vivid in New York than in any other American city. The explanation is simple; the colour of the square depends entirely upon the ratio of the Mexican, Indian, Puerto Rican or Negro to the general population."†

†Goldberg, B. *Procedures in Tuberculosis Control* Philadelphia, 1934.

These obvious facts can be verified in every mixed community. There are inherited factors which predispose certain races to succumb to the tubercle bacillus. Belonging to a particular race means that one has inherited habits of food, living, types of work, modes of response to environment. Inheritance of disease susceptibility is certainly a product of not one but several factors.

After the second world war the Western world woke up to the fact that the gravest tuberculosis problem lies not in the cities of Europe and North America, nor even in the devastated areas of Poland and Yugoslavia. It lies in Africa, East of Suez, India and Indonesia. A mix-up of populations was taking place. Primitive peoples were quitting the villages, using the bus and motor car to move to cities, work in mines and factories. Invariably their new environment and standard of living was different, and probably inferior to what they were used to at home. These new migrants into urban life faced the same problem as the Irish boy from Connemara, or the girls from the Outer Hebrides a generation ago, when they sought employment in Liverpool or Glasgow. Not only did they encounter the TB germ probably for the first time, but their habits of feeding underwent a big change. They worked at unaccustomed tasks, for longer hours, in a novel and testing environment. Now the same thing is happening all over Asia and Africa. In the course of two generations the Irish and Highland immigrant to the cities has learned to adapt to urban life and nowadays has less tuberculosis than his father or grandfather. But the African who migrates five hundred miles from his village to work in the mines has still to undergo that subtle process of acclimatisation. His former life moved at a leisurely tempo. Now he goes into the unknown modern world which is so fiercely intolerant to anything primitive.

The problem of tuberculosis today is not entirely one of infection, nor yet response to infection. It is a summary of different factors in the life of a human being called upon to make a tremendous adjustment in the space of a few years.

2

Even before the second world war, the Association was uncomfortably aware of the tuberculosis problem overseas, and sent Dr. Noel Bardswell, a leading specialist, to undertake a survey in Cyprus. This island, originally Greek, has had its population mixed with every race of the Mediterranean – Turks, Phoenicians, Saracens and even travelling Normans on their way to the Holy Land. The island has shaken down to a pair of cultures – Greek and Turkish. Bardswell found that the Cypriot population was tuberculin positive about six to eight per cent, and commented "I have been impressed by the frequency of the introduction of tuberculosis from outside the island, especially from Greece." Yet for a period at least, Cyprus had been singularly free from the disease but when immigrants came from the European mainland they brought a more serious type of infection. One result of the Bardswell report was the opening of the Jubilee Sanatorium, and tuberculosis dispensaries in Nicosia, Larnaca and Limassol. Cyprus is a typical example of how a rural people living in scattered communities, encounters invaders carrying the tubercle bacillus. In long, cold winter evenings the people were thrown together in small houses and in a few years the greater part of a family might be wiped out. Then once again the village could settle down, so to speak, to an epidemiological repose with few active cases. The work of the TB clinics was of paramount importance. Unknown cases could be traced and the spread of infection prevented. The National Association had taken in Cyprus one first small step in the fulfilment of its Empire obligations. In Cyprus the Survey was a stimulus to official action and Dr. Charles Bevan developed an excellent scheme before he was tragically killed during the political trouble.

Professor S. Lyle Cummins, was commissioned to undertake a tuberculosis survey in Burma, then a British Colony. This distinguished professor had a long record in the Army Medical Service and as a professor in the Welsh National School of Medicine and with him tuberculosis was a life passion. He made a general survey of a wild country of fourteen million people, half a million concentrated in Rangoon. He examined patients up and down Burma. He estimated the TB death rate as over 300 per 100,000. He had a curt word to say about environment "I do not propose to discuss housing beyond saying that the central part of Rangoon would be all the better for being burnt to the ground." Lyle Cummins found positive tuberculin reactions of twenty-six per cent in children under ten and sixty-one per cent in the older children. Prisoners in jails showed positive reactions of over forty per cent. Since Burmese and Indians always boil their milk before use, it seemed to him certain that the infection was of the human bacillus. His sad conclusion was that the cities and villages of Burma were far behind the West in their anti TB organisation.

3

Meanwhile on the slopes of Mt. Kilimanjaro, the highest mountain in Africa some seventeen thousand feet above the sea, Dr. Charles Wilcocks was working among the Chagga tribe, as a colonial medical officer. He was medical superintendent of the Kibongoto Hospital near Moshi, half way up the mountain, where a small antituberculosis unit had been set up in 1927. There he opened a laboratory and calculated that the incidence of tuberculosis in Tanganyika Territory was about 11 per 1,000, and there were some seventy-seven thousand actual cases among seven million people. The disease was locally called 'kifua-kikuu' and a simple bout of coughing might produce a terrifying haemoptysis from which death could follow in a few minutes. With a wretched official grant of £150 he opened a mud and wattle hospital with twelve beds. Patients cooked their own food over a fire in the traditional way. The doctors had nothing but a stethoscope, a microscope and a few drugs – among them, strangely enough, sanocrysin – the gold injection mentioned earlier. The treatment was largely ineffective, yet enough patients recovered to make the doctors feel that much more could be done. Mountain dispensaries were organised in the mission hospitals and sometimes a patient could be isolated in a separate hut near his village. Charles Wilcocks had an assistant Norman Davies who in 1932 returned home for leave with a pneumothorax apparatus, while Dr. Wilcocks provided his portable X-ray machine. Soon they were training African dressers to give artificial pneumothorax refills, and before long, ten dispensaries were in operation in a seventy mile stretch, the sessions being weekly or monthly, rain or fine throughout the year. The artificial pneumothorax refill was given anywhere – a honeysuckle hedge, or on the counter of a village shop. More buildings went up to accommodate up to a hundred patients, with one X-ray dark room and a primitive operating theatre. The X-ray itself was called *Haya haya, Wangaeli* because that was the name of the man who drove the car. Power was obtained by putting the engine into top gear and running it at 30 miles an hour (with the vehicle stationary). Presently more complicated chest operations were attempted, but routine artificial pneumothorax therapy was the mainstay. Soon this remarkable unit on Mt. Kilimanjaro had a large X-ray set and patients were accepted from anywhere however advanced their disease.

Patients would come up to Moshi by morning train, have their refills and return home the same day. Eventually the Government replaced that haphazard collection of buildings by an up-to-date sanatorium at Kibongoto. Meanwhile tuberculin tests of schoolchildren showed a declining rate of infection – a proof that the clinical work was actually removing some infection from the community. Asians as well as Africans came from as far off as Zanzibar, Mombasa and Nairobi, even Kampala.

A new chapter opened for Dr. Norman Davies (who by now had succeeded Charles Wilcocks) when streptomycin and PAS became available. Other physicians in the colonial territory were repeating the pattern of work at Kibongoto and a full antituberculosis scheme was being built up. Gradually the methods changed, but not the basic policy, and by 1956 with only 230 beds at Kibongoto, Norman Davies managed to handle over fifteen hundred in-patients during the year. In 1958 the National Association awarded to Dr. Norman Davies its Sir Robert Philip medal for this highly original work.

4

In 1944 the Association asked Dr. W. Santon Gilmore to undertake a survey in Trinidad and Tobago which have a population of about half a million. Dr. Gilmore had wide experience as a tuberculosis physician in Yorkshire. He established the fact that at the end of the last century the Trinidad tuberculosis death rate was about 274 per hundred thousand, but in 1946 this had fallen to 104. In the towns most adults were tuberculin positive. In Trinidad the intake of food is low. In the cocoa and fishing industries the labourers would consume less than 2,500 calories per day, and among asphalt workers no more than 1,400 calories. Moreover this diet seriously lacked calcium, vitamins and iron. Gilmore considered that these wretched levels of subsistence might explain the high tuberculosis death rate. He sketched proposals for the future, a sanatorium, rehabilitation schemes and financial assistance.

Towards the end of 1949 several officers of UNICEF (United Nations International Children's Emergency Fund) visited Malta to find out how the rising generation could be helped to recover from wartime hardships. Dr. Hans Jacob Ustvedt, chief physician of the Ullevaal Hospital in Oslo, carried out this investigation. He had already been responsible for BCG vaccination campaigns in Poland and elsewhere. He decided that the best policy would be to offer free BCG vaccination for all Maltese children between one and eighteen and to those over eighteen who desired it. An organisation called the International Tuberculosis Campaign (supported by Denmark, Norway and Sweden) would supply all the material, and the Government of Malta would finance the personnel. In 1950 the Chief of Mission arrived in Malta. He was a Norwegian, Dr. Andreas Weidemann, Medical Officer of Health for the city of

Trondheim, who had vast experience of tuberculosis work at home. The Health Department had already arranged meetings for doctors at which the Government Chest Specialist, Dr. V. Zammit Tabona, explained the idea behind the proposal. At the opening the Governor, the Archbishop, and Prime Minister undertook that the campaign would have their backing. Parish priests were visited individually and asked to explain the importance of vaccination. Schools and classrooms were used, the press was supplied with information and local radio stations gave talks. One small town with a population of over 12,000 people was chosen. Its inhabitants mainly followed heavy manual work in the naval dockyard and the standard of living was that of the average skilled labourer. The proportion who presented themselves was high. Out of 4,600 between one and eighteen years some 2,600 came for the tuberculin test, and 347 were positive. That is, about 15.2 per cent had primary tuberculosis infection and were, in a sense, already vaccinated. Thereafter all the main centres of population were visited and some 50,000 people tested. The BCG vaccine used in this survey came from the State Serum Institute in Copenhagen, being sent every week in insulated boxes, and it stood up well to the high temperatures. No vaccine sample older than fourteen days was used. A large number were vaccinated and only a tiny proportion had any complications. BCG vaccination has the power to change the tuberculin reaction of the individual from negative to positive in about six weeks. In the schoolchildren who went through this procedure the method was effective in 99 per cent.

We are now within an entirely different dimension – that of preventive medicine. BCG has been an enormous boon to tropical and sub-tropical countries.

In this story we have already come across Dr. Halliday Sutherland one of Philip's Edinburgh pupils who had become a tuberculosis specialist in London. Sutherland was a life-long lover of Spain who put his Spanish experiences into several popular books – which had nothing to do with tuberculosis. After the second war Halliday Sutherland revisited Spain and investigated the work of the national *patronato*, the semi-official organisation in charge of tuberculosis. He found that in 1939 the total number of sanatorium beds was 5,607, whereas ten years later this had increased to 17,000. Meanwhile the tuberculosis death rate had fallen from its high peak during the civil war – 129 per 100,000 – back to the pre-war peak of 112, this despite crop failures, droughts, and wartime devastation.

During this immediate post-war period, the International Union underwent a burst of expansive activity which has made the Union a powerful force in the modern campaign against tuberculosis. The Union had been set up as one of the hopeful features of the visionary time that followed the first world war. Its founders were Professor Léon Bernard of the Paris Faculty of Medicine and Sir Robert Philip, who gathered around them leading specialists from Europe and some from America. The first conference of the Union was held (1920) in London with Sir Robert Philip in the Chair. During the inter-war period, the Union held a conference every second year, and it was only after rejuvenation that followed the liberation of Europe from the Nazis that it really began to play a significant role.

Professor Etienne Bernard – an academic successor of Léon Bernard (but no relative) – became Secretary-General. Apart from his high reputation as a clinical specialist in tuberculosis and head of an important service at the Hôpital Laennec, Etienne Bernard is an orator in the classic French tradition, whose brilliant addresses at each International Conference have a very wide scope and are generally enjoyed. He is the son of Tristan Bernard, a leading writer of comedies and renowned for his wit. His son Etienne has inherited his father's magnetism and his travels over the world have brought the Union into great prominence.

After the second world war, steps were taken to make the Union truly international and it now includes some one hundred countries of the world. It appointed as its first Executive Director a talented man, Dr. W. Gellner, who set up research committees and regional conferences, and established a pattern which was to be developed by his successor, Dr. Johannes Holm, under whose management the Union spread its influence throughout the world, especially the world of the Far East where tuberculosis flourished among the eighty per cent of the world population who live in India, Indonesia, China and Japan. The International Union has now become truly international, as its founders dreamed. It holds large conferences every second year but has a number of 'Regions' – Middle East, Far East, Africa, South America, etc., etc., where specifically local problems are discussed. The Union also organises international research upon an increasing scale.

At first sight, it might be thought that this carefully planned organisation had arrived when there was no longer need for it, owing to the decline of the disease. This, however, would be an unduly narrow view, since the Eastern lands have not so far shared the decline in the disease which Sir Robert Philip so confidently predicted. Even in 1950 the WHO estimated that in the world a whole five million had died from tuberculosis. The International Union is proving that tuberculosis still keeps its place as a scourge of humanity which is almost universal and by no means eliminated.

The tiny seed of organisation which first germinated in Britain nearly a century ago, is now a mighty tree.

5

The problem of using sophisticated modern drugs in undeveloped countries had become challenging. Tropical governments have strained health budgets. If Western medicine were to become part of their medical organisation the use of an expensive drug like streptomycin would have to be curtailed. In 1955 the World Health Organization (in collaboration with the Indian Council of Medical Research, Madras Government, and British Medical Research Council) set up a research centre in Madras. The centre had a clinic and laboratory and a large domiciliary service. It had also 100 sanatorium beds and a statistical department. The first aim was to compare, a hundred TB patients living at home in the poorer sections of the city, with one hundred patients admitted to the sanatorium. This investigation gave a surprising result. Poor diet, poor housing, little rest, little nursing, irregularity of taking medicine – all these were found to have little or no influence on the patient's progress as compared with the powerful effect of drugs (isoniazid + PAS). In India, and other places with appalling hygienic backgrounds, it seemed that the drugs were more important than the transfer of the patient to healthy conditions. The same research formula was applied to home contacts. Were these people in their home conditions (more horrible than any European slums) more likely to develop tuberculosis than sanatorium patients? Here again the answer was clear – and surprising. All contacts with a case of TB are at serious risk in their home surroundings, but when the actual patient is being treated by drugs, even though he does not leave home, the risk to his contacts is greatly reduced. The contacts did not seem to be in any greater danger – provided they were being treated with the two drugs. This finding in the Madras Survey reversed the classic teaching based on Western experience. It has produced a revaluation in the handling of tuberculosis in the East.

Dr. Wallace Fox, an experienced and imaginative member of the Medical Research Council staff, took a leading part in the Madras Survey and was awarded (by the NAPT) the Sir Robert Philip gold medal.

The antituberculosis scheme in India was directed by a remarkable man – Perakath Verghese Benjamin, a Christian born in Travancore and educated at the Madras medical school where he took his degree in 1921. He chose tuberculosis as his professional vocation and in 1930 came to Europe and took his diploma at the Welsh medical school under Professor Lyle Cummins, and also visited the Scandinavian countries, then the centre of preventive ideas. Returning to India, Benjamin became Medical Superintendent of the Union Mission Sanatorium at Arogyovaram (place of health) in South India, and here for 10 years he established a first-class sanatorium regime. Benjamin attained such a reputation that he was soon noticed in New Delhi and became technical adviser to the Tuberculosis Association of India and later to the Government. His influence throughout the sub-continent was enormous, and also throughout eastern Asia he established training courses, set up conferences, advised on expert committees, started an Indian tuberculosis journal. His greatest achievement was the National Tuberculosis Institute in Bangalore where courses are given to doctors, nurses and others as students come from all over the east. The emphasis here was on prevention and Benjamin's vision and intense will-power made a revolution in the outlook. He received many honours and distinctions – from Great Britain, from India itself. He was the first Sir Robert Philip medallist of the National Association. This remarkable Indian got his way by a combination of charm and energy, and the support he received from the Minister of Health, Rajkumari Amrit Kaur, has been enormously beneficial to India.

6

Before the second world war, the phrase 'Maginot Line' – that powerful system of fortification which was supposed to protect France from invasion – came to be the perfect symbol of delusive security. A similar mode of thought prevailed among some tuberculosis physicians when they proposed that a strict cordon should be thrown around Britain to keep out cases of TB from abroad. This became a serious issue during the 1950s when immigrants from the West Indies, India and Pakistan were forming colonies in such cities as Birmingham, Wolverhampton and elsewhere. Our Ministry of Health decided that the elaborate controls that would be needed to keep out tuberculous people would be unwise and unnecessary. This was the right policy. The modern world is a shrinking world, and barriers between countries are no longer practicable if physical and mental equipoise is to be preserved. The system of segregation is wrong whether applied to any group – or even to a whole country. A better solution was found although it came later when much damage had been done.

In India the British High Commission arranges for all Indians who apply for 'work vouchers' to be medically examined in several centres, New Delhi, Bombay, Calcutta and Madras, where necessary with an X-ray. Dependants can also be included. The Indian immigrant who comes to one of our Midland cities seems to bring with him the same liability to develop tuberculosis as he would if he remained in his native village, that is, the Indian tuberculosis death rate is approximately double that of Britain. Breakdowns from tuberculosis occur not at the beginning of the immigrant's sojourn here, but after a year or so. The disease is not usually acquired before entry. It is unfortunately a reaction to the very different conditions of living and working that the Indian immigrant has to meet in a Western city: a new climate, longer hours, overcrowding, and a strange diet – although nowadays there are numerous Indian shops where the immigrants get food they like. Our tuberculosis clinics are well equipped to handle those who develop tuberculosis, and no alarmist attitude is justified.

7

After the war the Association developed an original scheme of scholarships and fellowships for doctors, nurses and health workers from various countries of the Commonwealth and Empire. This received the blessing of the Colonial Office and Colonial Governments. The Chief Medical Officer of the Colony would choose the candidates, who were given free travel and had their salaries continued for the three or six months of the scholarship period. The Association would look after them in the UK, arranging the postgraduate course that seemed most appropriate. Candidates were required to promise that they would go back home and use the knowledge they had gained. These scholarships do not represent a diploma course, they are more in the nature of a fresh experience for those who have already some knowledge. They are also a big intellectual stimulus for young men and women who have come for the first time to Europe. Over twenty-five years some 320 such scholarships were awarded. The Association has been gratified by the goodwill these doctors and nurses feel, and contact is kept up when they return home. There are also fellowships, valued at £500, to help more senior doctors to come to this country for postgraduate training.

It might be thought that the break up of the Empire would bring an end to this promising scheme. The opposite is the case. Many former Colonial countries keep up their relationship with the Association and send their scholars, even after Independence.

Chapter 16

Farewell to Trudeau

WE can look back to that milestone, it was more than a hundred years ago when Edward Livingstone Trudeau, under sentence of death from tuberculosis (with a stay of execution for twelve months) decided to enjoy his final year of life in the Adirondack wilderness. As we know, he never forsook that fascinating locality. Trudeau lived in the open air day and night to an extent that the Victorian age thought positively devilish. The village of Saranac Lake grew to a city. There he watched helplessly while his own son died of tuberculosis and nearly all the friends of that first winter. Trudeau lived to be sixty-seven, a world honoured leader, one of the first in America to follow the open air method, and today where he built his famous sanatorium a bronze statue overlooks the valley he loved so well. He had enormous personal influence over his patients, and the principle he taught was that the way to conquer tuberculosis is through acquiescence.

Then in December 1954, the Trudeau Sanatorium finally closed its doors to tuberculous patients. What had happened? Was the open-air tradition exploded? Is the sanatorium to be a mere historical memory? Like the carbolic spray, the wooden stethoscope, and the horse ambulance? The doors of Trudeau are closed, but for years the argument remained open and the world was doubting whether open-air sanatoria were necessary at all. Cases of TB are rarer, and we have outgrown the idea of pine forests. Patients are treated in ordinary hospitals provided proper precautions are taken. Forest-cure resorts distant from the cities are no longer essential, in fact they are impossibly inconvenient. Yet – the sanatorium principle of rest and acquiescence does hold a value in medicine even today. Bodily and mental repose remains Trudeau's therapeutic legacy. We can pass a gentle salute to his greatness. Whatever the open-air sanatorium may become, the name of Trudeau is an inspiration.

One reason for the closing down of Trudeau was a change in economic environment. After his death in 1915 the State of New York, the wealthiest in the North American commonwealth, had built several handsomely equipped modern sanatoria to provide treatment virtually free of cost, whereas the Trudeau institution remained a private one which charged fees.

2

But open air is still the medium in which the lungs operate. The oxygen we breathe has a lumbering partner – nitrogen – present in a much greater amount and virtually inert. This nitrogen acts as a dilutent. An animal breathing pure oxygen would die as rapidly as it would in pure nitrogen.

Nowadays however the idea of fresh air connotes a new and sinister element – that of atmospheric pollution. Sulphur dioxide from power stations is a chemical poison which so far, the law has not been able to eliminate. The ultra-violet rays of the sun convert this into sulphur trioxide which joins up with droplets of moisture and becomes an irritant to the lungs.

Aerial hygiene began with a simple experiment. The test performer washes out his mouth with a culture of a harmless but tenacious microbe (B. proteus) and then shouts across the room. In the course of this vocal exercise droplets of moisture are propelled into the air, and the test microbe can be detected forty feet away. A trained opera singer can project air to an even greater distance. Thus the air in any inhabited place is full of moisture and microbes from human lungs and human throats. Room air may contain fifteen bacteria-carrying particles per cubic foot, although filtration can reduce this by three quarters. The viruses are an even more dangerous component of aerial infection, for viruses are light and resistant and can migrate long distances. Pessimists say that when the last human being has gazed upon the ruins of St. Paul's from London Bridge, viruses will be ready waiting to inhabit the earth.

We shall have to take aerial hygiene more seriously in the future. It would be impossible to live permanently in an artificially controlled atmosphere. The air seems dead and there is no proper relationship between what we breathe and the excretion of moisture from our skin. Sir Leonard Hill showed, half a century ago, that what is wrong with stagnant air is not merely its carbon dioxide, but the fact that it does not perform its normal function upon the human skin. The movement of a fan restores the sense of comfort, even though the oxygen content remains unchanged. We are only beginning to explore the significant chapter in human experience which originated with Trudeau. Aerial hygiene includes the prevention of tuberculosis and many other respiratory diseases, like virus pneumonia, and numerous allergies caused by breathing pollen or dust, but also the most sinister of all, that of nuclear particles which we do not know how to control. Even primitive folk, decreasing in number, such as hunters and fishermen will now have to consider aerial hygiene, and gregarious man who lives in groups will require a new type of crowd medicine. The oxygen and nitrogen in the air enveloped round the earth will not change, but the localised atmosphere of the factory and the bedroom can be highly injurious. A London street may contain sixty-three airborne bacteria per cubic foot, while in an Underground station the figure could be one hundred and fifty-two. How are we to get the active oxygen, without germs or viruses, or nuclear radiation? The future task of the MOH and hygienic engineer is going to be vital.

3

During the 1950s the scope of the National Association changed. Chronic bronchitis, much neglected, came to the front. This illness is so much more common in Britain than in Europe that it has been called the 'English disease'. Above the age of forty, bronchitis is responsible for ten per cent of the male sickness rates: twenty-five million working days are lost in a year, and 30,000 die of it. Here is an illness which takes the position that tuberculosis occupied in the early years of the century. The respiratory system still remains the 'Achilles Heel' of modern man. Water-borne diseases like cholera we have learned to control: we eliminate malaria by killing the mosquito: but air infections are hard to prevent in overcrowded situations. The total area of one person's internal lung surface – all vulnerable and continuously bathed by the air we breathe – is at least fifty square yards, an astonishing expanse, equal to the quarter of a tennis court. The climatic influence in disease is sometimes exaggerated, but here is an illness where temperature, winds and rains do really matter. The death rate from chronic bronchitis is a hundred and fourteen in Manchester, in Eastbourne it is fifty. A prevailing wind may concentrate smoke upon particular districts and so increase the smoke-laden air droplets which contain sulphur dioxide. Air which erodes the stonework of Westminster Abbey bears hard on the human lung. The victim of chronic bronchitis has a wretched cough, worse in the morning or after exertion, and he cannot properly expel the residual air from his lungs, so that 'trapping' of air causes further shortness of breath which is aggravated by bronchial spasms. He feels he cannot ever breathe in enough air – yet to no human being is oxygen more precious. The bronchitic patient dreads the winter and hangs over daily weather forecasts. He feels the cold, loathes climbing a hill, running for the bus, and fears equally a draught or a stuffy room. He has constant anxiety whether he will be fit enough to go out tomorrow and this makes him a poor performer in industrial life. And each winter season he gets into a justifiable panic lest his death knell be sounded through a sudden smog. These depressing features of chronic bronchitis were well known to the doctor fifty years ago and recent research merely clarifies what has long been obvious. It is tempting to feel that until the smoke nuisance has been cured there can be no help for these patients, but the unfortunate bronchitic cannot bide twenty years for the air of his town to become smoke-free, or two centuries for the south-west wind to change its course. Through individual therapy, properly directed breathing exercises (they are not appropriate in every case), the correct drug treatment of minor respiratory illnesses in the winter, the decline in morale can be checked. The doctor can relieve symptoms, prevent relapse, stave off disaster and often forestall a breakdown. In an elderly patient such efforts can add years to the patient's life. For the bronchitic patient cigarette smoking is not only the most harmful factor in his disease, but the only one he can personally control.

4

Granite hewers in Aberdeen, Kaffir gold miners on the Rand, makers of fine glass in the Five Towns of England, these gnarled and often romantic figures conceal the grave spectre of dust disease. Constantly inhaling silicates makes them forgetful of its consequences, makes the world forget too, and twenty or more years later comes the final chapter of the sad story, when the middle-aged man permanently disabled by shortness of breath is quite unable to to work.

Silicon, the most ubiquitous, the hardest, the sharpest element in nature has a devastating and capricious effect on the lung tissues. Not only diamond dust, granite dust and gold quartz are dangerous: and apart from silicon, new trades introduce new dust diseases under that general title, pneumoconiosis. These are now covered by compensation schemes which contain a large element of preventive medicine. In 1930 a new form of dust disease – asbestosis – was recognised, and we are painfully learning that asbestos is used in many forms such as the brake lining of cars. There is also the disease caused by fluffy particles of cotton and wool, a condition called byssinosis. Fortunately we are learning our lesson and there is more control of the hard dust diseases, especially in coalminers. In 1956-1957 some 13,000 men in Britain were examined by pneumoconiosis medical panels, and about half received compensation. They came from an astonishing range of trades – coalmining, pottery, metal grinding, steel dressing, metalliferous mining, etc., etc. 'Good housekeeping' in the foundry can achieve something, but masks though useful in theory are as unpopular as nurses' masks in hospital wards. Gradually the heavy steel industry will be carried out in modern plants where newer techniques can virtually eliminate risks, but there are still numerous small foundries where the danger is as great as ever it was.

A fitting symbol of these men whose lungs are metaphorically being turned into stone would be of Henry Moore's grotesque figures. No one who has ever seen one of these pathetic fellows will ever forget the man who is so breathless that he sits all day in an armchair, with not enough vital energy to poke the fire.

We can say a heartfelt farewell to Trudeau – the man and the sanatorium – but his idea is an immortal part of preventive medicine.

Chapter 17

The Final Decade

BY the year 1950 the National Association was half a century old and had survived with triumph over the difficult conditions of the post-war period. The rise in tuberculosis which followed the war, and the extreme shortage of beds, were now being overcome. The techniques – medical and social – by which the community can conquer this illness were well understood, and the paramount need to look outside Europe, towards those countries east of Suez where tuberculosis is the number one medical problem, were being grasped.

The decade between 1950 and 1960 is interesting nonetheless for several activities which, but for the war, would almost certainly have been started earlier. Mr. Albert J. Mantripp was now Secretary and took a large part in health education. The Association opened a Scottish branch in Edinburgh and was fortunate enough to get Mrs. Margaret Stirling, whose name has appeared before as a pioneer of tuberculosis in the Highlands, to become Chairman. She fulfilled this office with great charm and skill, and, when eventually she retired, she was succeeded by Dr. W. M. Murray, with Mr. David Turner as Scottish Director. The Scottish branch conducts activities of its own on broadly the same lines as the parent body and has established itself as a force in Scottish Preventive Medicine.

Another and very different activity of these post-war years was an enquiry into the psychological background of the tuberculous patient. It was conducted by Dr. Eric Wittkower (afterwards Professor in McGill University, Montreal) and when his findings were published in a volume (1949) entitled *A Psychiatrist Looks at Tuberculosis* it was probably the first occasion in modern times in which the disease had been scientifically examined with modern techniques. The book was introduced by Dr. John Rickman, a well-known psycho-analyst. Dr. Wittkower had collected his material on the personal interview technique. It emerged that the tuberculous patient erects 'psychological defences' to his illness and that in time this becomes for the unfortunate individual even more menacing than the illness itself. Dr. Wittkower analysed the many personal attitudes which surrounded the patient – those of the physician, of the family, and the general reactions which came from the environment. To these the patient responds in many diverse ways; through hypochondriacal tendencies, child-like faith in the doctor, aggressiveness, etc., etc. and these modes of self-defence were as important in every way as the blood reactions to the bacillus. Dr. Wittkower probed much more scientifically than previous writers this emotional factor in the tuberculous patient's life which has been mentioned earlier in this book. For instance, he classified the patient's bouts of 'premorbid personality'. There are many insecure people, the rebellious, the 'self drivers' and the 'self drivers in reverse'. Such conflicts were the cause of harassment to the human beings who make up the mass of tuberculous invalids. The originality of Dr. Wittkower's book lay in applying these analytical methods to a disease which was previously considered nothing more than a bacteriological and toxaemic episode in the patient's life.

Then, in 1959 the Association published a handbook of the various methods of social rehabilitation which can be applied to the tuberculous family. This was written by Miss Margaret Coltart and Miss Elizabeth Harrison and it gave, ten years after the National Health Service had become law, what was available. The fact that in many geographical areas of the country the arrangements fell below ideal standards demonstrated how in this post-war period giant strides had been made towards some kind of social justice for the TB family, and if many could not yet obtain what they needed it was partly because the norm had been raised considerably above pre-war ideas.

In this decade the Association published numerous other reports, handbooks and summaries which represented the culmination of its teaching during the century, and as the year 1960 approached it was realised that the old NAPT must now reshape itself to meet a new world. Tuberculosis was now firmly under control through the Regional Hospital Boards and Local Health Authorities. The need for a 'pressure group' to stimulate progress was not so great as in the beginning of the century and the Association was settling down into a middle-aged condition of self-satisfaction with what had been achieved. There were even some who thought that the Association should now commit an act of hari-kari, a ceremonial suicide in the glory of sixty years of achievement.

However, the structure of the National Health Service prevented any such negative move. The old tuberculosis officers had now become chest physicians and their clinics (formerly called dispensaries) were being filled by patients whose diseases, although confined to the chest, had nothing to do with tuberculosis. Chronic bronchitis, lung cancer and asthma were being studied with a new kind of intensity. It was realised that chronic bronchitis alone, it was being called the 'English disease', causes deaths in a year almost equal to what tuberculosis did sixty years earlier. Also it was realised that functionally the heart is part of the chest in the sense that it functions inside the thorax. Also, in some ways, the rehabilitation problems of cardiac patients are similar to those which face the chest patient. It was decided that the Association should reflect this important change and, without abandoning tuberculosis, should take part in modern chest medicine.

It was realised too that not only the new chest physician with his nurses and social workers, but the chest clinics too had a stake in this important change. Legal difficulties would have prevented the NAPT from taking on these new interests in its old constitution. The change was made, and in 1959 the Association was restyled THE CHEST AND HEART ASSOCIATION.

2

That powerful and emotive phrase 'the conquest of tuberculosis' gave inspiration to a movement when it was very young. The crusade seemed glorious and the Holy Grail was certain of attainment.

Now, as we take a backward look, with the experience of sixty years, what may we conclude? It gives a sense of dismay to realise that we have not by any means completely conquered tuberculosis, or even fully unveiled its cause. Tuberculosis, is still common, still virulent. It is like a wild animal in the forest which lies in wait for any of us, and our success is more in the nature of a truce with the enemy: an interval in a cyclical struggle rather than the eradication of which some people speak too glibly. Tuberculosis, it is certain, was already on the decline a hundred years ago before Robert Koch discovered the bacillus, and what we have seen in our own day may be the end of the epidemic which followed the industrial revolution of the last century. This might seem a poor result for so much heroic aspiration and conscientious effort. Surely, we say, the efforts of Villemin and Koch, the teaching of Robert Philip has had some effect?

It is a fact, or rather a paradox, that although our weapons are stronger than ever (the new drugs for instance) the virulence of the germ is still over-powering, under favourable conditions. It still has its waxy capsule, its power to produce different families, and its ability to generate toxins. Nor do we fully understand the phenomenon of resistance. What makes one brother safe in a tuberculous family and causes the other to be struck down? Sometimes it seems just an application of the old harsh law that to him who hath shall be given. To those who have a good natural resistance we give drugs. To those who have no resistance at all we can give little.

Yet tuberculosis has taught humanity many valuable lessons. The study of this disease was the beginning of epidemiology. The open-air revolution represented man's liberation from his habit of self-enclosure. He opened the windows and regarded the open-air life as something to be desired. He learned that ventilation, the use of sunshine, are natural and therapeutic. Even the sanatorium lessons of rest in a temporary retreat from life had a meaning, for the curative art is not so rich in resources that we can neglect this primary fact. We may smile now at the fanaticism of the open-air devotees, yet if we read the Victorian novelists we can recall the stuffy bedrooms, excessive clothing, over-feeding, and we can be grateful that we live in the post-sanatorium era.

Then again tuberculosis provided the beginning of chest surgery and in the 1930s it was the principal reason for a chest operation. Old Jimmy Carson's prophesy that the human chest could be opened and the lungs collapsed, required nearly a hundred years before anaesthesia and antiseptics made this procedure possible. Artificial pneumothorax opened a new chapter in our knowledge of the mechanics of breathing. After the new drugs appeared in the 1940s chest operations for TB became rarer as the emphasis of chest surgery moved over to lung cancer. Then children with tuberculous hips and spines who came in such numbers from the slums of our cities were the first to benefit from what is now called orthopaedic surgery. Sir Robert Jones and Dame Agnes Hunt were curing hideous deformities and almost eliminating the need for amputation simply by a process of rest and splinting in the open air.

3

If there is criticism to be made of those heroic pioneers in the antituberculosis campaign, it is that they did not go far enough or allow their principles sufficient scope. Between the wars, housing was neglected and nutrition in its scientific aspects hardly applied. BCG vaccination succumbed to a wave of panic and took 20 years longer to be accepted than was necessary. Sanatorium physicians who had their patients under careful observation for months and years did not make use of the newer methods which psychiatry had introduced and, looking back, it is astonishing to realise how little Europe realised that tuberculosis is indeed a global, rather than national, problem, and like malaria, plague and cholera, it is a big part of tropical medicine.

Although tuberculosis is now declining in every country of the world, the great killer is not dead, but his bluff has been called and we know how to forestall his attacks and to some extent neutralise his virulence.

Yet tuberculosis, it seems to me, would be of limited interest (except to the specialist) apart from the human beings who have suffered and still suffer today. Theoretical studies do not carry us far enough. Some may criticise the title of this book – *Requiem for a Great Killer* – but a requiem is an opportunity for recalling disaster, not entirely in sadness, for on this occasion there is a message of hope. In the long history of the disease countless people were cured, many found in this crisis of their lives a rude shock which was a new beginning. They pass, this long procession, down the ages, and they turn to greet us. These ex-tuberculosis sufferers are telling us – "We were good patients, we taught ourselves to acquiesce and to control the disease, and we taught the medical profession to study us as individuals and not to let their science become frozen in theory." The theme of the requiem is this: the patient is more vital than the disease. The modern TB patient is in a much more fortunate situation than his counterpart in the 1930s. Today he will receive his treatment by pills while continuing to work at a job. No longer is he regarded as a pariah. There is a strong element of hope in every case and patients can look forward to complete recovery without tiresome refills or major operations. Here is the theme of the requiem. It needs still the faith of the passionate few who will resist the brute pressures of germ toxins and human ignorance.

THE END

INDEX